Women Ageing

Changing identities, challenging myths

Edited by
Miriam Bernard,
Judith Phillips,
Linda Machin and
Val Harding Davies

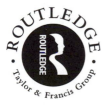

London and New York

First published 2000
by Routledge
11 New Fetter Lane, London EC4P 4EE

Simultaneously published in the USA and Canada
by Routledge
29 West 35th Street, New York, NY 10001

Routledge is an imprint of the Taylor & Francis Group

© 2000 Miriam Bernard, Judith Phillips, Linda Machin and Val Harding
Davies
Typeset in Times by
Prepress Projects Ltd, Perth, Scotland
Printed and bound in Great Britain by
Biddles Ltd, Guildford and King's Lynn

British Library Cataloguing in Publication Data
A catalogue record for this book is available
from the British Library

Library of Congress Cataloging in Publication Data
Women ageing : changing identities, challenging myths/edited by
Miriam Bernard ... [et al.].
     p. cm.
  Includes bibliographical references and index.
  ISBN 0-415-18943-8 (hbk) ISBN 1-415-18944-6 (pbk)
  1. Aged women. 2. Middle aged women. 3. Aging – Social aspects. I.
Bernard, Miriam
HQ1061.W636 2000   00-055360
305.244–dc21.

For Sue
In appreciation of the support and friendship you have given each and every one of us over the years

Contents

Illustrations

Figures

Tables

Contributors

Miriam Bernard (BA, PhD) is Professor of Social Gerontology and Head of the School of Social Relations, Keele University. Before joining the academic staff at Keele in 1988, she worked with older people in the voluntary sector as Research Officer for the Beth Johnson Foundation. Her research interests are primarily oriented around the development of new/healthy lifestyles in old age and she has a particular interest in the lives of older women. She has co-edited *Women Come of Age – Perspectives on the Lives of Older Women* with Kathy Meade (Edward Arnold, 1993) and *The Social Policy of Old Age – Moving into the 21st Century* with Judith Phillips (Centre for Policy on Ageing, 1998). Her most recent book is *Promoting Health in Old Age: Critical Issues in Self Health Care* (Open University Press, 2000).

Pat Chambers (BA, PGCE, MA) joined the School of Social Relations, Keele University, in June 2000 as a lecturer in social work. She came from the Centre for Healthcare Education at University College Northampton, where she had been responsible for the development of a part-time undergraduate degree in gerontology. She previously worked at Stockport College of Further and Higher Education for 15 years, teaching a range of social care and social work courses; it was during this time that she obtained an MA in gerontology from Keele. Her academic interests include gender and ageing, disability, involving older people in research and biographical research. She is currently completing part-time doctoral research on the experience of later life widowhood.

Gillian Granville (BA, MA, RN, RM, RHN, CPT) is Research and Development Manager at the Beth Johnson Foundation, a national organisation based in Staffordshire which aims to develop and research innovative practice with women and men over 50 years of age. Until 1993, she was a health service practitioner and worked with women experiencing menopause. During that time, she also obtained her MA in gerontology from Keele University. She is currently completing part-time doctoral research examining women's mid-life experience of menopause and ageing. Her other research interests include feminist research methodology, gender and the life-course and intergenerational approaches to understanding ageing.

Val Harding Davies (BEd, Dip. Counselling, MA, Cert. Counselling Supervision, Advanced Diploma) is Director of Counselling Courses at Keele University. She is also a practising psychotherapist and counselling supervisor. After a period of early employment in industry, she qualified as a teacher and subsequently became a lecturer in the Youth and Community Department of Manchester Metropolitan University, where she taught psychology and interpersonal relationships. Val is currently engaged in part-time doctoral research examining trainees' experiences of counselling training. With a colleague from Durham, she is also editing a book on this topic.

Linda Machin (MA) has been actively engaged in research and practice related to bereavement since 1979. She has a number of publications including *Looking at Loss* (Pavilion, 1998) and *Working with Young People in Loss Situations* (Longman, 1993), both of which are practitioner-focused books. Linda founded a counselling service – Bereavement Care – which serves the North Staffordshire area. Since becoming a lecturer at Keele University in 1990, she has continued to focus on issues of bereavement and is completing her doctorate, which explores the nature of the diverse range of response to loss.

Judith Phillips (BA, Dip. Soc. Sci., MSc, CQSW, PhD) is Senior Lecturer in Social Work and Gerontology and Director of the Social Work Programme at Keele University. After a period of employment as a social worker, she completed her doctorate at the University of East Anglia (UEA), examining the admission process into private residential care, where she then became a research associate and a lecturer in social work. Her current research interests include working carers, housing and older people, family and kinship networks and older offenders. Her recent publications include a co-edited book, *The Social Policy of Old Age – Moving into the 21st Century*, with Miriam Bernard (Centre for Policy on Ageing, 1998) and *Broadening our Vision of Housing and Community Care* (1999).

Mo Ray (BA, MSc, CQSW, Dip. Geron. PhD) graduated in 1988 from the Open University and subsequently qualified as a social worker, receiving her Masters degree in 1990 from the University of London. She has worked in a variety of social work posts focusing on work with older people, and also spent a year working at the Royal College of Nursing (in partnership with the Alzheimer's Society), authoring standards of care for people with dementia who live in care homes. She has recently been awarded her doctorate from Keele and currently works as an Associate Lecturer for the Open University and as a Research Fellow at Keele, working on a European Commission-funded project exploring intergenerational relations in families. When time permits, she continues to practice teach social work students.

Julie Skucha (BA, MA, PhD) entered higher education as a mature student at the age of 27. After completing research at Keele on women part-time workers' transition to retirement, she undertook doctoral research on the process of becoming a mature female graduate. She has worked as a Lecturer in Sociology and Women's Studies at the University of Wolverhampton and is currently Research Fellow in the Centre for Research into Quality at the University of Central England.

Acknowledgements

As with any book, there are very many people whose contributions we would wish to acknowledge. First and foremost, we thank the many women with whom we have come into contact through our research and practice. They talked willingly and openly to us and we were privileged to share parts of their lives. Although we have not been able to use the words of everyone, all your 'voices' have influenced our thinking, both professionally and personally. To those who also took part in focus groups, pilot studies and who read and gave us constructive criticism about our research and writing at various times, a big thank you.

Particular organisations also facilitated and sponsored our research and writing and we would especially like to thank Keele University, the University of Luton, the Open University, the Pre-Retirement Association, Bereavement Care and the Beth Johnson Foundation. We thank Vintage for permission to quote from *Object Lessons: The Life of the Woman and the Poet in Our Time* by Eavan Boland.

The contributors wish to acknowledge the support of the editors and all the authors involved with this book – reflections on the fun and frustration involved in this process can be found in the concluding chapter!

The editors also wish to thank a number of individuals who assisted greatly in the last stages of the book's production: Margaret Bernard for her careful editing and useful comments on the introductory and concluding chapters and Sue Allingham for transforming a medley of drafts into a coherent whole, patiently and good humouredly as ever. Our appreciation goes finally to our editors at Routledge, Heather Gibson and, subsequently, Edwina Welham.

Foreword

There could scarcely be a topic of more intellectual, social and economic importance in the early twenty-first century than the focus for this book: the way in which women experience the process of ageing in British society. Older people are of increasing importance to the vitality, stability and development of this society. Women are crucial to these.

The simple reason for this is demography, in which there has been a dramatic change during the later part of the twentieth century. In 1901, one person in twenty was aged over 65; by 1998, it was one in six. Similarly, in 1901, only one person in 100 was over 75; by 1998, it was one in fourteen. This dramatic shift in the age balance of the population begins much earlier than any conventional definition of 'old age' and affects women and men unevenly because of differing survival rates. At the present time, women begin to outnumber men from the age of 50 onwards. By age 89, there are three women for every man.

So, from early middle age, women become an increasingly dominant group in demographic terms, and therefore an increasingly central force in a society which must learn to make full use of the talents of its older population if it is to flourish. But how do women experience this process? Does it feel like a process in which the crucial role of older women is recognised and valued?

The varied chapters in this book explore these themes from different angles – the scholarly, the personal and the political. Rooted in social science perspectives, the book draws widely on those theoretical frameworks that can illuminate women's experiences of ageing: feminism, life-course development and critical gerontology. The evidence base is also varied, blending autobiography with other types of social science data reflecting, as the editors say, a desire to move away from the 'add women and stir' approach. In so doing, the book reflects upon methodology – how properly to study older women's lives – not just upon the substance of its topic.

To an extent, the book places women where they have always

conventionally been– in the home and caring for families – and explores how ageing maps onto domestic roles and relationships. To locate women in the domestic is in itself to explore both the private and the public. Twenty-five years ago when, in my own work, I began research on what was then called 'informal caring', I realised rapidly that women's apparently private lives raise profound public issues. Women were then – and to an extent still are – running a support service for their sick and frail relatives, which was at least as large in scale as the official health service, provided their labour was properly accounted for. The private can be not only a public issue but also a highly political one when viewed in this light.

Alongside these well-identified topics, the book also tackles less explored dimensions of older women's personal lives, such as bereavement and the menopause. The focus is on lived experience and completely avoids any sense of women as victims of biological and social fate. Women appear in this book as people who, for the most part, cope well with change and adapt to new circumstances. They also appear as people whose lives are by no means confined to the domestic. They are people whose identities are deeply invested in paid work, sometimes in very demanding jobs, and who actively embrace education and the new horizons that it can open in later life. Some of the authors themselves attest to the importance of education and work in their own experiences as older women.

So, do older women feel that our society recognises and values their importance to social and economic health? Not yet this book tells us. But, in raising the profile of these issues in a sensitive and imaginative way, this work should contribute to moving the consciousness of our fellow citizens in the right direction.

Professor Janet Finch
Vice Chancellor
Keele University

1 Women ageing

Changing identities, challenging myths

Miriam Bernard, Pat Chambers and Gillian Granville

Introduction

The authors of this book are women who have been, and in many cases still are, associated with what was formerly the Department of Applied Social Studies at Keele University and is now part of the School of Social Relations. We have academic interests and professional backgrounds in gerontology, social work and counselling, and many of us have taught both undergraduate and postgraduate students. While the book reflects these professional interests, it also draws specifically on the research that we have all undertaken on various aspects of the lives of mid-life and older women. The book is concerned with understanding better what ageing is like for women and has been developed around a series of key themes and issues. In particular, we are concerned with the ways in which women construct and reconstruct their identities in mid-life and beyond and how this changes. This involves consideration of the multiple identities which women develop and of the negotiations and renegotiations which occur as women deal with particular transitions or circumstances in their lives. We also hope to challenge some of the myths which have grown up around women's traditional roles and expectations of ageing, showing how the reality of our lives during the second half of the life-course is still shaped and constrained by a variety of external pressures. We uncover not only the commonalities and similarities between mid-life and older women but also some of the variation and diversity relating to ethnicity and race, class, disability and sexual orientation. The concluding chapter explores the range of strategies that women adopt in managing these changes to their own lives and the possible responses which society now needs to make in terms of both policy and practice.

The opening chapter provides an overview and introduction to the theoretical perspectives, key themes and issues pursued in subsequent chapters. All the major chapters are framed by an adherence to what might be described as a critical, feminist, life-course perspective. This perspective draws on a number of theoretical strands but has, at its heart, the desired intention to make more visible the ordinary lives of ordinary women as, in this instance, they grow older. We argue that the body of literature and research that we have to date has led either to the experiences of mid-life and older women remaining invisible or to an inevitable pathologising of their situations. This chapter also presents some of the thinking and principles which underlie what we are trying to do: the theory and the methods associated with our approach. The central chapters are concerned much more with illustrating the key themes through empirical research and/or professional experiences. In order that readers are clear about how we are using particular terms, we also discuss definitions of key words and phrases. Finally, we give a brief overview of the succeeding chapters.

Rethinking theory

Everywhere we turn these days, we are confronted with reminders about growing older. As women in particular, we are bombarded daily with media images designed to stave off the physical signs of ageing: wrinkle-smoothing creams; hair dyes; tooth-whitening products, to say nothing of the boom in cosmetic surgery (Belcher, 1999). Both the popular and the academic press frequently carry articles about the impact of our ageing population on the economy, on health and welfare services and on intergenerational relations (Kaye, 1999). However, we still know comparatively little about how we, as women, view our own ageing and about the day-to-day experiences of growing older in an increasingly ageing society. The way society is constructed, alongside myths and notions about women's natural roles and predispositions as carers and mothers in particular, sets up tensions and ambiguities in thinking about, and reflecting upon, these issues. Central to this are concerns about our own identities as women. The visible signs of ageing and the 'ageist standards of appearance' (Ann Gerike, 1990: 41) to which we are subjected make manifest these tensions.

All adult women are, whether we like it or not, ageing women. Yet, although the growing academic interest and the increasing 'coincidence of age and gender' in the literature (Diane Gibson, 1996: 433) is to be welcomed, there is still comparatively little empirical research, certainly in a British context, which attempts to make visible the lives of mid-life and older women. The little we do know is predominantly focused on heterosexual, white and often middle-class women (Miriam Bernard, 1998), with minority ethnic women, women with other sexual orientations, poor women, disabled or differently abled women being some of the most marginalised and neglected groups (Meredith Minkler, 1996). We need, therefore, to be aware of the dimensions which bind us all together as women, but also alert and sensitive to the rich variety of differences and experiences among us (Colette Browne, 1998). Some sense of this variety can be culled from the increasing numbers of academic texts which address the lives of mid-life and older women (Ellen Gee and Meredith Kimball, 1987; Katherine Allen, 1989; Diane Garner and Susan Mercer, 1989; Sara Arber and Jay Ginn, 1991, 1995; Miriam Bernard and Kathy Meade, 1993a; Barbara Turner and Lillian Troll, 1994; Browne, 1998; Linda Gannon, 1999; Jenny Onyx *et al.*, 1999). Together with 'popular' volumes written either by older women themselves or which contain transcripts and conversations with middle-aged and older women (see, for example, Susan Hemmings, 1985; Mary Adelman, 1986; Janet Ford and Ruth Sinclair, 1987; Jewish Women in London Group, 1989; Jean Shapiro, 1989; Germaine Greer, 1991; Suzanne Nield and Rosalind Pearson, 1992; Ruth Thone, 1992; Betty Friedan, 1993; Hen Co-Op, 1993, 1996; Dorothy Rowe, 1994; Charmian Cannon, 2000), this growing body of writing is testimony to the fact that, as Browne (1998: 269–70) observes:

> Aging women, demanding corrections to ageist and sexist myths, are insisting that their voices be heard and respected rather than ignored or patronized.

Although we strive, in this book, to contribute further to this body of literature and to address the points that Colette Browne raises, it is important to note that our premise is that no one existing theoretical perspective has a monopoly when it comes to trying to explain or to understand women's lives: we draw on a variety of intellectual traditions and theoretical developments to inform the work presented here.

Above all, we have a continuing commitment to a life-course approach, in tandem with insights from feminist perspectives and critical gerontology. We first advocated such an approach early in the 1990s, arguing that it: 'is crucial to our understanding of the situations which confront women as they age' (Bernard and Meade, 1993b: 9). Within a life-course approach, the importance of a life span developmental perspective is one which has taken a while to become recognised. However, both we and other academic colleagues around the world have argued that such a perspective is vital if we are to understand better the interplay between the individual and the broader society in which we live (Bernard and Meade, 1993a; Browne, 1998; Gannon, 1999; Onyx *et al.*, 1999; Matilda White Riley and John Riley, 1999). Critical gerontology and feminism also have much to offer to the study of ageing in general and to the lives of mid-life and older women in particular. To show how these differing perspectives inform successive chapters, each is discussed in more detail below.

Perspectives from critical gerontology

Social gerontology has been undergoing something of a sea change in the ways in which we think about ageing and old age for both women and men – and indeed in some of the sources of data that we use. In recent years, these issues have come together under the umbrella of what is now labelled 'critical gerontology'. Ruth Ray (1996: 675) defines critical gerontology as: 'a critique of the social influences, philosophical foundations and empirical methodologies on which gerontology as a field has been historically constructed'. Critical gerontology has grown out of the broader critical social science movement and draws on at least three strands of work evident in gerontology's historical development (Achenbaum and Levin, 1989; Achenbaum, 1997).

First, it has its intellectual origins within the political economy perspective: a perspective associated in North America with the writings of people such as Carrol Estes and Meredith Minkler (Minkler and Estes, 1991) and in Britain with Townsend (1981, 1986), Walker (1981, 1982) and Phillipson (1982). Political economy perspectives have been very influential in getting us to look critically at how growing old is experienced, maintaining that the welfare state has effectively transformed ageing into a dependent status rather than providing opportunities for self-determination and continued participation in everyday social life. Although this perspective began to raise crucial questions about ageing for women, initially at least, it largely concentrated on class rather than gender as its main analytical orientation (Arber and Ginn, 1991).

A second strand emphasises an increasing concern with the uncertainties surrounding ageing. Drawing on work from the humanities (notably history, philosophy and ethics), this addresses the potential for loss of meaning in the lives of people as they age (Moody, 1992). This is linked with, and influenced by, insights and contributions drawn from post-modernism which suggest that now, more than ever, we ought to look at ageing and old age as a fundamental part of the entire human existence rather than spending our time and effort trying to stave it off or to substitute things which disguise or assert youth-oriented values (Molly Andrews, 1999).

The third and final strand is gerontology's 'rediscovery' of the importance of biography in extending our knowledge and understanding about both individual and shared aspects of ageing (Johnson, 1978). Anne Jamieson and Christina Victor (1997) contend that this tradition is well established in Britain and, in Bill Bytheway's words (1997: 14), 'this cataloguing and enumeration of our past … is the way in which the past contributes to our sense of age'.

By bringing these strands together, it is possible to see that key issues affecting the lives of mid-life and older women have come under increasing scrutiny from the critical gerontology perspective. Conventional topics such as education, employment and income, health and well-being, poverty and pensions, caring and social relationships are all being discussed in much greater detail. However, as Gibson (1996) notes, much of this still focuses on what is wrong with ageing and older women, how they are socially disadvantaged and what can be done to correct this. Older women are still considered as 'other' to older men, prompting Gibson (1996) to call for a less 'phallocentric' analysis of women in old age. Approaches which emphasise women's biographies and the need to hear women speak for themselves are going some way towards answering this criticism. We now have, for example, a growing body of literature which exhorts women to redefine and re-examine our identities as we age in an effort to achieve a more authentic mature self (see, for example, Hemmings, 1985; Ford and Sinclair, 1987; Greer, 1991; Friedan, 1993; Hen Co-Op, 1993, 1996). In very recent years too, there have been attempts to put what Meredith Minkler (1996: 470) describes as 'a human face – and a human body and spirit – on ageing and growing old'. This essentially humanistic orientation, embraced by many gerontologists now researching and writing about the post-modern life-course, stresses both the diversity and the multiplicity of lifestyles touched upon above – but also argues for the use of data such as literature and visual images to help us to understand and explain the meanings and significances that we attach to ageing and old age.

Two particular issues arise from this. First, gerontology in general, and critical gerontology in particular, has made the study of ageism central to its concerns. This is fundamentally important to our understanding of the experience of ageing for women and is an issue which many of our central chapters address. The possession of negative attitudes based on age is one facet of the key social oppression that we now recognise as 'ageism'. As Bill Bytheway and Julia Johnson (1990) have shown, the impact of ageism is such that it can generate and reinforce a fear and denigration of the ageing process itself. Along with racism and sexism, ageism manifests itself in all sort of ways in our society: in the vocabulary that we use, in visual imagery, in institutional policies and in discriminatory structures and practices (Butler, 1980; Johnson and Bytheway, 1993). None of us are immune to the impact of ageism and, for women in particular, it often intersects with sexism to produce particular pressures on us in terms of ageing and our physical appearance (Susan Sontag, 1978). As Colette Browne (1998: xxvi) also argues, ageism hits women harder than men in a number of other spheres, 'leaving them with their financial, health, care giving, and social status seriously impacted'.

Not only is ageism rife among the population at large, we can also note that it is alive and well among those who care for older people in professional capacities (Olive Stevenson, 1989). The radical American feminist Baba Copper (1988: 60) goes even further and accuses women of what she terms 'woman-to-woman' ageism: younger women can and do exploit older women, although the opposite is also true (Browne, 1998). These observations alert us to the tensions and complexities surrounding ageism and to some of the ways in which women are treated, and treat each other, in our society. One graphic illustration of the impact of ageism on women comes from the writings of Pat Moore (1986). At the age of 26, she decided to disguise herself as an 85-year-old woman in the hope that it would enable her to learn more about the ageing process and how the products that she was involved in developing as an industrial designer could be made more sensitive to the needs of older people. The 3 years that she lived as an old woman enabled her to document in detail the ways in which she was treated. This ranged from indifference and being short-changed by shopkeepers to verbal abuse and being assaulted and left for dead by a gang of youths. In a different cultural context, Sheila Green, a British nurse, found very similar attitudes being expressed when she repeated elements of this experiment (Sheila Green, 1991; Hope and Bernard, 1992).

Second, although theoretical writing and empirical research constitute particular forms of gerontological 'evidence', perspectives from the humanities have also demonstrated the benefits of complementing this with other, perhaps less conventional, 'data' in the form of literature and visual images which are particularly helpful in illuminating what ageing means for women. One illustration of this, which graphically portrays the struggles some us have with our own ageing, comes from the memoirs of the Irish poet Eavan Boland (1996). She writes about womanhood, nationhood, places and times in her life and about the ways in which traditionally silent women can find a voice through being the authors of their own poetry, rather than simply the objects of others' poems. She describes putting her memoirs together 'not as a prose narrative is usually constructed but as a poem might be: in turnings and returnings' (Boland, 1996: xiii). One of the 'turnings and returnings' that Boland deals with is ageing, and how difficult she found this to write about when younger. After talking to an older woman on one summer's evening in Dublin, she recalls how:

> I begin to make notes for a poem. I try to write it. As I do, I am aware of that split screen, that half-in-half perspective which is so connected with the act of writing… At some point I do what I have rarely done – at least not at such a preliminary stage of writing. I put down the pen. I leave my notes. I set aside the poem in the complete certainty that it will never be written.

(Boland, 1996: 203–4)

She goes on to dissect in detail what it is that has prevented her from writing this poem, concluding that it is nothing to do with either the suburb in which she lives nor with the Dublin hills behind it. Eventually, she writes (Boland, 1996: 206–7):

Where the women stand and talk – deep within that image is, I know, another image. The deeper image is that shadow, the aging woman, the argument that the body of one woman is a prophecy of the body of the other. Here, at the very point where I am looking for what Calvino calls 'that natural rhythm, as of the sea or the wind, that festive light impulse,' the exact opposite happens. I cannot make her real; I cannot make myself real. I cannot make the time we are happening in real, so that the time I fear can also happen... I sensed, hidden in the narrative distance between myself and this theme of aging women, some restriction, some thickening and stumbling... I could not write these women... that I could not write it was nothing new. What unsettled me was that – at some level I barely understood – neither did I feel free to imagine it.

That, as a young woman and a poet, she could neither experience this sense of what ageing is like nor indeed imagine it was, she found, most upsetting: 'I want a poem I can grow old in. I want a poem I can die in' (Boland, 1996: 209) she laments. Yet, years later in mid-life herself, she is now able to write:

That moment has come to me which was prophesied by another woman's body in a summer twilight years ago. I am older, less hopeful, more acquainted with the craft, more instructed by my failures in it. And once again there is a notebook open on the table by the window... I walk to the table. I sit down and take up my pen. I begin to write about a river and a woman, about the destiny of water and my sense of growing older. The page fills easily and quickly.

(Boland, 1996: 238)

Eavan Boland articulates for us just how difficult it is to recognise and acknowledge one's own ageing, as well as the alliances that one might develop with other older women. The value of such introspective commentaries is that they offer us one way of getting 'inside' the experiences of ageing (Achenbaum, 1997: 24). As women, we are having to deal with a great number of complex and often contradictory messages about who we are, what we should be doing and how we should be dealing with growing older. It is precisely these kinds of contradictions, complexities and ambivalences which, as authors of this book, we are attempting to address.

In sum, critical gerontology, although it may still be 'an aspiration rather than a body of knowledge' (Jamieson and Victor, 1997: 178), alerts us to some of the ways in which society continues to oppress us as we age. It argues that ageing issues and older people have been marginalised and ignored and it prompts us to question long-held and taken-for-granted assumptions and beliefs about old age, old people and the ways in which we and society respond to them. It also calls into question some of the traditional theories and methods that we have used to study ageing and old age, and is both about explaining how oppression and injustice occur and affect people as well as about attempting to make the voices of oppressed groups such as older women and black elders heard. Here, it is clear to see that these ideas resonate very strongly with feminist perspectives. Indeed, both Minkler (1996) and Achenbaum (1997) argue that feminist perspectives have integrated and invigorated critical gerontology by stressing the gendered nature of ageing and growing old and by getting us to look critically at what has been called 'the social construction of women's marginality in old age' (Walker, 1987: 9).

Feminist perspectives

Although there is not the space here to provide a detailed historical overview of feminism, it is important to flag up a number of features about its development that influence our own work and current concerns. In particular, we call attention, first, to the difficulty of defining exactly what feminism is. Second, it is important to note the way in which feminism has moved from being an active grass roots movement into the 'academy', and how this has, in turn, led to debate between the various feminist perspectives which now exist. Essentially, these perspectives divide into the 'traditional' ones, which date from the beginning of the second wave of feminism in the 1960s and 1970s and include liberal, radical and Marxist/socialist schools, and the 'contemporary' perspectives, which developed in the 1980s and 1990s and have their origins in psychoanalytical and post-modernist/post-structuralist discourses.

Some writers define feminists as those who identify themselves as such (Shulamit Reinharz, 1992), whereas others emphasise feminism's links with particular theories as to the causes of the social injustice experienced by women (Maggie Humm, 1989). In this context, feminism becomes a political label, indicating support for the aims of the women's movement and the struggle against all forms of patriarchy and sexism (Toril Moi, 1989). More recently, some writers prefer to use the label 'feminisms' in order to convey, more accurately, the multiple theoretical perspectives that feminism now encompasses (Sandra Harding, 1991; Ray, 1996; Sandra Kemp and Judith

Squires, 1997). Others lament the fact that contemporary society has forgotten what feminist ideas and goals are (Judith Evans, 1995), whereas bell hooks's (1984) belief that feminism's central problem is its inability to reach consensus or to accept definitions that could serve as points of unification is still relevant today. A clear and agreed definition of feminism is therefore difficult to find. It thus helps to turn to the historical development of feminism in order to illuminate more clearly some of its influences on our own work.

The development of feminism

The first point to stress here is that feminism is not a single, unified approach. There are now a great many variations, but from the 1970s to the 1990s it became common to divide them up into categories to highlight the contrasts and similarities between them (see, for example, Hester Eisenstein, 1984; Juliet Mitchell and Ann Oakley, 1986; Rosemarie Tong, 1989; Evans, 1995; Kemp and Squires, 1997). It has also been conventional, within much of the British and American literature, to distinguish between two waves of feminism; the first wave spanning the period from 1830 to 1920, and the second from the 1960s to the present day.

'First-wave feminism' was founded within a classic civil rights perspective and its focus was on campaigns for women's enfranchisement and the extension of civil rights to women (Evans, 1995; Kemp and Squires, 1997). In Britain, it is considered by many to have come to an end when women achieved the vote, and the period from the 1920s to the 1960s is viewed as a dormant or silent time for feminism (Ann Oakley, 1981; Kemp and Squires, 1997). 'Second-wave feminism', meanwhile, is commonly thought to have begun with the publication, in 1963 in America, of Betty Friedan's book *The Feminine Mystique*. Throughout the 1960s and 1970s, the movement was characterised by extensive and active networks of women's groups and by campaigning at grass roots level for changes in women's circumstances. As noted elsewhere (Bernard and Meade 1993a), the movement at this time tended to reflect the interests and concerns of mainly younger, white, middle-class articulate women. The situation of women in the home, the division of labour, child care and reproductive roles and issues around women's sexuality were of prime concern (see, for example, Shulamith Firestone, 1971; Sheila Rowbotham, 1973; Oakley, 1974).

The 1960s to 1970s was also the period when the 'traditional' approaches to feminism began to be articulated. Here, we can identify three major approaches: liberal feminism, radical feminism and Marxist/socialist feminism (see, for example, Tong, 1989). Crucially, for our purposes, all of them were concerned with articulating the causes of oppression suffered by women and all saw women as a unified category and as 'other' to men. Patriarchy, capitalism and the public/private dichotomy were central concerns.

Liberal feminists argue that women's oppression lies in their lack of civil rights and in their poor educational opportunities. The goal is to achieve equal rights with men, not by changing the structure of society but by reform and legislation to improve women's position. By contrast, the emergence of radical feminism in the late 1960s saw patriarchy, through its social, political and economic institutions, as responsible for the social injustices suffered by women (Humm, 1989). A key theme in radical feminism has been the control of women's bodies by men, for example through sexuality, reproduction, motherhood and rape (Browne 1998), and radical feminists have been vocal in encouraging women to take control of their bodies. However, radical feminist theory came under considerable criticism during the 1980s because of its overtly reductive accounts of female sexuality (Kemp and Squires, 1997).

Marxist/socialist feminism also believes that women are oppressed by society's structures but that it is the interlocking of capitalism with patriarchy which is the primary cause. Socialist feminists linked class domination with patriarchy, arguing that in order to understand women's experiences and needs it was necessary to analyse the interaction between the public mode of production and the private realm of reproduction. Women's needs and experiences, in both the public and the private sectors, should be part of the socialist agenda. Integral to this is the raising of consciousness to counter the silence of oppressed groups. In the context of this book, it is important to record that socialist feminism was responsible for first drawing our attention to the unpaid domestic labour of women and to women's segregation in employment into low-paid jobs (Browne, 1998).

However, we also have to note that the concerns of mid-life and older women were notable by their absence during much of first- and second-wave feminism. Certainly, in Britain, this was not part of the feminist agenda (Hemmings, 1985; Zelda Curtis, 1989; Arber and Ginn, 1991). It is really only since the 1990s, a period sometimes referred to as the post-feminist era (Kemp and Squires, 1997), that ageing has begun to be addressed within a feminist framework. This contemporary period also marks the retreat of feminism into the academy (Evans, 1995; Kemp and Squires, 1997) alongside renewed concerns that feminism, as in the first wave, is coming to be dominated by white, middle-class women speaking on behalf of others. As a counter to this, contemporary socialist feminists, for example, now tend to place much greater emphasis on the multiple layers of oppression that they see women as being subject to – and particularly the ways in which patriarchy and capitalism interlock with class, gender and racial domination to structure and organise society. They see no single or universal category of 'woman', but make a commitment to trying to understand the experiences of women of colour, working-class women, disabled women, poor women, lesbian women and old women as well as white, financially privileged, heterosexual women (Toni Calasanti and Anna Zajicek, 1993; Browne, 1998). Contemporary radical feminists, meanwhile, tend to focus more on particular issues, such as pornography, family violence, assault and rape and, importantly, on the collective group known as 'women' rather than on individuals. Catherine Mackinnon (1989), for example, suggests that radical feminist theory must define sexual reality on its own terms and argues for more empirical work to understand women's experiences. She believes that women do not seek sameness with men nor to dominate men: the issue here is not gender difference but the difference gender makes.

Psychoanalytic feminism, sometimes known as cultural feminism, believes in the creation of a separate women's culture, arguing that women have innate qualities which should be valued and claimed as their own. Carol Gilligan (1982) considers that the primary problems we face today are because women's values are not affirmed in a male-centred society. As with traditional feminism, one of the main criticisms of psychoanalytical/ cultural feminism has been its tendency to ignore differences within and between groups of women (Judith Butler, 1990; Evans, 1995).

Post-modern and post-structural feminists also contribute to the continuing debates about whether or not there is a single unified concept of 'woman'. They stress plurality rather than unity and are concerned that by declaring the existence of a universal 'woman' there is, by implication, a set of characteristics that make up that concept and which become the norm for that group. Moreover, too strong an emphasis on women as a group subject to power, repression or exclusion denies the possibility that oppression is not the same for all women. However, lest it seem as if post-modern feminists are abandoning the collective concept of feminism, their argument is rather that they wish to deconstruct the ideas, to scrutinise them and to reconstruct the elements. It has also to be noted in turn that some feminists are critical of post-modernism and are uncomfortable with the belief that there is no one identity. This issue, and the associated theorising around it, dominated contemporary feminism in the 1990s in sharp contrast to the more practical, grass roots concerns of the traditional feminists of the 1960s and 1970s.

Contemporary feminists are concerned also with the exploration of issues of race and ethnicity, and the development of what has been termed a 'cultural politics of difference'. Feminists working in this field criticise Western feminism as being inattentive to race and ethnicity and as failing to recognise the power differentials among women. They categorically reject any shared identity based on women's experiences of oppression but, instead, argue that what they name 'white' feminism has prioritised sexual difference above others (Beasley, 1999). There is concern that most of the issues faced by black and minority ethnic women are different from those of white women because the relationship between the two is fundamentally structured by racism. bell hooks (1984:18) is highly critical of the racism that she sees in feminism and is convinced that:

> …women from exploited and oppressed ethnic groups dismiss the term (feminism) because they do not wish to be perceived as supporting a racist movement; feminism is often equated with white women's rights effort.

More recently still, the debate about a cultural politics of difference has led to attempts to move away from gender, race and ethnicity towards even less distinctive groupings that enable those who are invisible and do not fit neatly into them to be more adequately considered (West, 1993). Caraway (1991) suggests that we need 'multicultural coalitions' without domination and advocates the importance of knowing about where and why an individual is situated in society. This current emphasis on the importance of situating ourselves in society leads naturally into a consideration of biographical and life-course perspectives as one means of uncovering further what ageing is like for women.

Biographical and life-course perspectives

As with traditional and contemporary feminisms, many existing psychological models and theories have been criticised for failing to take account of ageing or of mid-life and older women's experiences. Thus, the growing interest in a life-course perspective and in life span developmental psychology is to be welcomed because, essentially, 'it does not write women off just because of their particular age, class, race or sexual orientation' (Bernard and Meade, 1993b: 9). Jamieson and Victor (1997: 181) further argue that a life-course perspective is 'best viewed as a map of orientation, suggesting important points to look out for on the road to an understanding of ageing', and that adherence to such a perspective provides a basis for biographical studies.

The life-course of individuals has been described by Leonie Sugarman (1986) as a sequence of events and experiences in a life from birth to death which are influenced by personal states and encountered situations. She and others (Bond *et al.*, 1993; Slater, 1995) also suggest that a life span developmental approach has much to offer the study of ageing. In particular, it stresses that the potential for development extends throughout life and that development is multidirectional and can occur on a number of different fronts. This approach also recognises the individual and the environment as influencing and being influenced by each other, such that individual ageing is situated within a wider societal context. The attraction to the study of ageing of a model of psychological growth and development throughout life is clear, particularly because, as Slater (1995) reminds us, substantial numbers of us will be embarking upon these 'not well-trodden' paths. However, while it may offer a useful organising framework for such study, some writers argue that its theoretical basis and its examination of the relationship between agency and structure still needs further development (Bury, 1995).

Until recently, human development has most commonly been constructed as a series of identifiable stages or phases, the most well-known and frequently cited being the eight-stage theory of Erik Erikson (1980). Daniel Levinson and his colleagues (1978) also developed a staged model of the life-course, consisting of a series of steps alternating with transitional phases. Interestingly, although his model was based on empirical work with men, he does discuss distinguishing features of the mid-life transition, one of which is the masculine–feminine polarity. He suggests that men in early adulthood emphasise their masculine side and women their feminine side, but that in mid-life the balance is redressed.

Similarities can be found between Levinson's work and Erikson's model, but both have been criticised on a number of counts: for their limited empirical work; for the unreliability of retrospective life-course accounts; and for the generalisations which are drawn, particularly when gender differences are not acknowledged. Even very recently, Sherry Willis and James Reid (1999: 279) have been critical of the lack of attention in mid-life literature to issues of gender and gender equality, commenting that: 'Many of the studies of normative development during middle age have used samples of only men'.

A central concern of the life-course approach revolves around identity and personality: in our case, what it means to be a woman in general, and an ageing woman in particular. Within the psychoanalytical tradition, the work of Carl Jung is particularly relevant to our study of ageing 'because of its conceptualization of changing priorities across the adult life span, which influence the balance between conscious awareness and unconscious influence' (Biggs, 1993: 20). It recognises the potential of people to adapt so that what is unacceptable at one age may be acceptable at another; it holds out the possibility that, as people age, they continue to develop and come to know themselves better. Here, we can draw parallels with some contemporary commentators on the interaction between identity and the social worlds that we inhabit over the life-course. From a sociological basis, Anthony Giddens (1991), for example, argues that the transformation of modern day-to-day social life has such a profound effect that the individual 'self' has to become more reflexive. Throughout the life-course, therefore, people develop greater understanding of themselves, which they are able to use to manage changing external circumstances. Although Giddens does not specifically write about ageing, he does acknowledge the impact of feminism and the ways in which women need to understand themselves and their self-identity. His work has also been influential in wider debates on the development of social identity across the life-course.

Richard Jenkins (1996: 3–4) defines social identity as 'a characteristic or property of humans as social beings'. It involves individuals making sense of who they are as well as who other people are, and it refers to the way in which individuals and collectivities are distinguished in their social relations with other individuals and collectivities. Jenkins suggests that identities have become more public in the consumer society, both for the individual and for groups. He believes that the theorisation of social identity must concern the *relationship* between an individual unique identity and that of a collective shared identity, arguing that the two are intrinsically linked. Furthermore, he makes an important distinction whereby individual identity emphasises difference, while collective identity is about the similarities that members share. He also asserts that identity has to be validated by those with whom we come into contact, stressing the importance of the *interface* between self-image and public image. Although Jenkins does not say so, it is possible to see links here between the sociological interpretation and the psychodynamic tradition, when Jung speaks of the interaction between conscious awareness and unconscious influence.

It is also important in any consideration of social identity to acknowledge the seminal work of Erving Goffman (1969). Goffman is particularly concerned with the way that individuals negotiate their identities, maintaining that individual identity is generated in the relationship *between* the self-image and public image (Jenkins, 1996). He considers that the individual has a frontstage public appearance that is presented to others and a backstage private one in which the embodied self can be free of the anxieties of presentation. It is in the backstage space that the individual can rehearse the public face. There is, however, little gender analysis in Goffman's writing, although he did consider sex as a fixed presentation of self to the outside world. Moreover, his theorising sits less comfortably within a post-modern analysis and within the more current emphases on the role of social masks and masquerades as applied to ageing and identity (Featherstone and Hepworth, 1991; Kathleen Woodward, 1991; Ephrat Tseelon, 1995; Biggs, 1999a).

Individual identity formation and development, together with deliberations about social identity, are key aspects of a life-course perspective. Yet, with some notable exceptions (for example, Gilligan 1982), gender and age have featured comparatively little as a focus for study or theorising, aside from an acknowledgement that a consideration of 'adult life' is a much needed corrective to the overemphasis on earlier phases of the life-course and the problem of age-based definitions (Jamieson and Victor, 1997). Jung (1968), however, claimed that women in mid-life gain easier access to the masculine side of their nature and become more aggressive, with a parallel occurrence happening in men as they develop feminine features of gentleness and caring behaviours. The work of anthropologist David Gutmann (1987) and of Bernice Neugarten (1968) also lends support to the idea that as women age they become more authoritative and assertive and better able to follow their own wishes. Other writers have challenged these notions, while Terri Apter (1995) highlights the dilemmas of being a mid-life woman, arguing that ageing women are now much more active in fashioning their identities and goals.

In addition to these disputes, one particular danger of a life-course perspective is that it can be seen to contribute to the pressures on us all to create an ageless society which potentially diverts attention away from its oldest members (Jamieson and Victor, 1997; Andrews, 1999). Although we would concur with the belief of Molly Andrews (1999: 315) that this denies people 'the real gift of age', we do not think that the two are mutually exclusive. We need the ability to see old age and old people as part of our own futures, while maintaining an interest in, and concern with, the process of ageing itself. One way in which it is possible to do this is through biographically based studies of ageing and old people.

Biographical approaches overtly acknowledge the importance of life-course experiences in shaping the present. Valerie Yow (1994: 168) defines biography as: 'the account by an individual of his or her life that is recorded in some way, by taping or writing, for another person who edits and presents that account'. This is not simply the recording of a testimony, but rather an interaction between the interviewer and the interviewee with distinct echoes and parallels with feminist research methodology. Biographical work has always been important to the women's movement both because it allows the voice of women to be heard and because it 'provides an opportunity for the woman reader and the woman writer to identify with the subject' (Reinharz, 1992: 126). This is particularly important when researching ageing and older women who, as we have already argued, are mostly either invisible or problematised. For women, biographies help to uncover a lifetime of 'experience; knowledge; passions; and decisions' and 'they help the whole person emerge from statistics or the distancing of differing generations and perspectives' (Bornat, 1993: 42). James Birren (1996: ix) has also suggested that the widespread interest among researchers in life histories is:

> ...due to a belief... That something important has been left out of our scientific knowledge generating system in its studies of adult change and aging. It is becoming increasingly clear that what has been omitted are the experiences of growing old and being old.

Biographical and life-course perspectives are then a necessary complement to the more scientific tradition, but, as we shall see in the following chapters, each has its part to play in the search for a better understanding of what ageing is like.

The impact of these perspectives on our own work

In the context of this book we, as authors, both relate to and take from the above perspectives a number of themes and points which inform our own work. First, in terms of our personal experiences, it is important to acknowledge that we were all teenagers or young women during the flowering of the second wave of feminism. Undoubtedly, we have all been affected, to greater or lesser extents, by the associated changes apparent at this time in terms of widening educational opportunities, control over women's reproductive cycles, abortion legislation, changes to both the private and public domains of work and the sexual division of labour, and the movement for equal pay among other things. Second, as our professional, academic and personal lives continued to develop, we have lived with, taught about and researched aspects of women's experiences, which have been informed by many of the writers and commentators referred to in the above discussion. In particular, our work has been, and still is, informed by concerns with:

- questions of social justice;
- making visible women's experiences through our own words;
- understanding oppression: its multiplicity and diversity;
- acknowledging the relationship and tension between the structural and the personal and between the public and the private lives of women;
- articulating the impact of economic and political power, institutions and knowledge on women;
- exploring what it means to be a 'woman': the commonalities and the diversity; the differences within and between;
- examining identity: its acquisition and development; its fluidity and changeability;

- expanding our understanding to include perspectives addressing race and ethnicity, age, sexuality, class and disability;
- developing a critically reflective, and self-reflexive, approach to both our own ageing and that of those around us.

In addition, we would all subscribe to contemporary calls for feminism to be more inclusive, for women's strengths to be recognised and for there to be coalition building which recognises plurality rather than stressing unity.

Although the work that we report on in succeeding chapters cannot address all of these issues all of the time, it does attempt to use feminist, gerontological and life-course approaches and concepts to illuminate something of what it is like to grow older and how that is experienced by mid-life and older women. As we ourselves have grown older, we have become more acutely aware of the ways in which the ageing process itself has been largely ignored, dismissed and denigrated. Although some feminists have, in recent years, begun to turn their attention to the lives of older women, this has largely concentrated on highly conventional, policy-orientated topics such as caring, institutional and community care, income and pensions, health and health services and housing and accommodation issues (Bernard and Meade, 1993a). While not denying the importance of these issues, the contributions included here constitute one small attempt to add a slightly different dimension to these discussions and to focus on how ageing itself intersects with, and shapes our responses to, contemporary social, economic, political and personal developments.

About this book

The phrase 'mid-life and older women' does not trip easily off the tongue, yet it is important that readers are aware of how we are using this term. We are critical of chronological definitions alone, subscribing, instead, to the view of Arber and Ginn (1995: 5) that:

> ...an adequate sociological theory of age needs to distinguish between at least three different meanings – chronological age, social age and physiological age – and how they interrelate. Chronological (or calendar) age is essentially biological, but needs to be distinguished from physiological age, which is a medical construct, referring to physical ageing of the body, manifest in levels of functional impairment. Social age refers to the social attitudes and behaviour seen as appropriate for a particular chronological age, which itself is cross-cut by gender... In all three meanings – chronological age, social age and physiological age – ageing is gendered.

In the chapters which follow, ageing is therefore used in all three of these ways, although some meanings are more salient in some analyses than in others. For ease of understanding, we generally use 'mid-life and older women' to refer to women who are in their forties onwards. However, where appropriate, each chapter unpacks this phrase in an effort to draw out the three meanings of age as well as highlighting other bases for differentiating women, such as cohort membership, racial, ethnic and class dimensions, sexual orientation and the nature of particular disabilities.

This diversity is further captured by the range of research methods that our authors use to study women's ageing. Although qualitative approaches have long been associated with feminist work, and biographical research is now firmly part of both gerontological and feminist research practice, the position that we adopt here is one which stresses the appropriateness of method according to the questions that one is asking. Indeed, Reinharz (1992) clearly demonstrates the range of methods now encompassed by feminist researchers. Gerontologists too are increasingly subscribing to the view that we need both quantitative measurement and qualitative understandings alongside a continuing critique of the activities that we are researching and the ways that we are going about it (Arber and Ginn, 1995; Jamieson and Victor, 1997). Thus, the research reported on here ranges from focus groups to individual and group interviews, to highly quantitative surveys and to batteries of tests, inventories and scales. Some of our research privileges one method over another; others use multiple methods and, on occasion, limited longitudinal methods. Reflexivity and ethical issues are also key to all the work discussed in succeeding chapters as we are concerned to take account of the ways in which our own experiences, skills and values impinge upon the research process. Moreover, in the final chapter, we return to issues about research with ageing women and, alongside 'conventional' cross-sectional approaches, advocate the increasing use of longitudinal life-course approaches.

Thus, in the nine chapters which follow, we attempt to examine what the process of ageing is like for women and how this has an impact on identity and on the myths and stereotypes which surround us. We open with a trio of chapters which all, in varying ways, consider the role that paid work has in shaping and reshaping women's identities as they age. In Chapter 2, Julie Skucha and Miriam Bernard begin by challenging two popular myths relating to women's participation in, and exit from, the labour market. The first myth is that participation in 'women's work' (i.e. part-time, low-paid and low-status work) is primarily motivated by the desire to supplement the family income in order to purchase luxuries. The second concerns the myth that retirement is generally a period of comfortable leisure which women approach with particular readiness. Based on the findings from a mixed methodology study exploring the pre-retirement needs of part-time women workers over the age of 45, this chapter seeks to deconstruct these mythical images. The findings in fact reveal that mature and older women workers have high levels of job satisfaction and attachment to the worker role. In exploring the transition from employee to retiree, this chapter also considers the most appropriate forms of support that women may need at this phase of their lives.

Judith Phillips then takes up some of these issues in Chapter 3, in which she explores the experiences of mid-life women who are trying to balance both paid and unpaid caring roles. As labour market changes increasingly require women in the workplace, and job flexibility enables them to take greater advantage of such opportunities, more women will be tempted back into paid work. However, existing research and writing on this issue is limited and myths abound, including the assumption that 'caring' comes naturally to women, that this identity is central to women's existence and is reinforced through gender socialisation, and that women's expressive nature is adequate preparation for coping with the stresses and pressures of paid caring work. Research also tends to proceed from the assumption that (female) working carers are a homogeneous group, that care giving will inevitably result in problems in employment, that women will substitute care for employment if they have to and that, in the end, it is simply a matter of balancing roles. The chapter challenges these myths, arguing that 'juggling' rather than 'balancing' best characterises the situations of these women, and that much additional research needs to be conducted before we can adequately determine how policy and practice can best be reoriented in order to assist working women in both their paid and unpaid caring roles.

Work, too, is central to Chapter 4, but, in this instance, it forms the backdrop to mid-life women's concerns about their own ageing. Val Harding Davies and Miriam Bernard explore the proposition that until we, as women in mid-life, fully understand and explore our own attitudes to ageing and old age, then we cannot work in ways that will be truly beneficial and empowering for the older women that many of us care for in our professional capacities. The chapter draws on the authors' exploratory research and counselling practice with professional women facing, and working through, a series of mid-life adjustments and transitions in their lives. It highlights both the fears and the creative possibilities that ageing holds for women, concluding with thoughts about how women can best be supported as they age.

We then look, in Chapters 5 and 6, at two contrasting areas of the mid-life experiences of women: menopause, which is a universal experience, and education, which is a very specific experience. In Chapter 5, Gillian Granville examines past and present approaches to understanding menopause and considers why it appears to be such a focus of attention for the medical profession and for feminists, but not the lived reality for many women themselves. Drawing on the results of a feminist inquiry with a diverse cross-section of 'baby boom' women, the chapter concentrates on menopause as a time of change for women, during which they come to recognise aspects of their changing private self while, at the same time, hiding this from the public gaze. Gillian's work clearly shows how many of us attempt to pass as younger women in order to maintain our identity and sense of who we are in the face of negative societal views of ageing.

Some women of a similar age also choose this time of their lives to enter education for the first time. In Chapter 6, Patsy Marshall reports on her biographically based qualitative research, which examines the motivations and experiences of women aged 50 plus attending two campus universities and the Open University. When women enter higher education at this age, they not only have to contend with society's myths about the proper role of 'grandmothers' but they also have to contend with their own myths and expectations that older people cannot learn, that only gifted people go to university and that women are 'better' at the arts than the sciences. This chapter explores the origins of these beliefs, the conditioning and socialisation of these cohorts of women and shows how they discover, or remain unaware of, the formative influences on their present educational and family lives. The chapter contends that, despite the difficulties these women face, this is often a particularly appropriate time for them to study for a degree.

With our concluding trio of chapters, we turn our attention to women's experiences of loss and to older age. Linda Machin focuses, in Chapter 7, on bereavement and loss, demonstrating how, to date, much theoretical work in this area has come from male, medical and pathological perspectives. She goes on to show that contemporary theoretical developments are now being driven by female researchers who are systematically seeking to establish the diversity of grief experiences, including the differences between women and men. This work provides a context for Linda's own research, in which she discusses how her own framework for understanding the diverse range of responses to loss is being empirically tested. Drawing on the results of continuing research with mid-life and older women, she examines how appropriate the framework is in helping us to understand how to work therapeutically with women in bereavement.

Conventionally, a key loss faced by many women in older age is the death of one's spouse. In Chapter 8, Pat Chambers explores the experience of widowhood in later life. She shows how existing work has led to a fixed model of widowhood which, she argues, is overly restrictive. A wealth of quantitative literature exists which tends to portray widowhood as a time of loss and as a discrete event which stands in isolation from the rest of women's lives. Her own research, utilising a biographical/feminist approach, begins to help us understand how older widows negotiate their lives in widowhood in the context of their whole life-course. It is important to see this transition in terms of 'new' roles rather than 'lost' roles, with widowhood as a potential beginning.

New roles also form a key theme of Chapter 9. In her exploration, Mo Ray adopts a feminist, grounded theory approach in order to elucidate the ways in which women in old age manage caring for, or being cared for by, a partner to whom they have been married for a very long time. Although there is already a considerable body of literature and research relating to caring and to long-term marriage, there is very little as yet which specifically links the two. Drawing on findings from her own research with long-married couples, she considers how disability (either her own or her partner's) has an impact on an older woman's identity and self-image. In particular, she shows how perceived continuities are used to construct current identities, how identities are readjusted as circumstances change and how this helps to explain ways in which strategies for managing change are used. In so doing, Mo Ray also challenges myths about women's natural propensity to, and lack of choice in, caring, as well as the view that very old women (and men) are an inevitable burden on the family and/or the state.

Our concluding chapter, Chapter 10, brings together the range of issues raised by contributors in relation to policy and practice and suggests that a new agenda for change is needed if both policy and practice are to respond adequately to the needs of women across the latter half of the life-course. Here, too, we review the limitations of this book and offer some reflections on the challenges and frustrations of the collaborative writing that we have undertaken.

Conclusion

Although we have brought together feminist, biographical and critical gerontological perspectives in order to explore what ageing is like for mid-life and older women, we are aware that we do not, and cannot, claim to represent the entire range and diversity of women's experiences. Much still remains to be done, and we therefore concur with colleagues who argue that a feminist age analysis is needed to provide a critique of the underlying premises and public and private policies that we use in conceptualising and responding to the needs of ageing women (Arber and Ginn, 1995; Browne, 1998; Onyx *et al.*, 1999). Such an approach recognises the interlocking of women's problems one with another and with each stage in the life-course and shows the multilayered routes of oppression that accumulate in women's lives. Together, Browne (1998: xxix) says:

Gerontologists and feminists must examine how to make these later years of life worthwhile and successful for today's and tomorrow's older women. [Finally] there is an important role for middle-aged and older women. They [we] must insist that their voices be heard and respected, not only by feminists and gerontologists but by society at large.

It is our hope that, in a modest way, we have begun to contribute to this developing process and accumulating knowledge base.

2 'Women's work' and the transition to retirement

Julie Skucha and Miriam Bernard

Introduction

The origins of this chapter lie in an exploration of the ways in which women may be helped in their transition to retirement through pre-retirement education (PRE). The research began by identifying the distinctive aspects of women's employment in their later working lives. This led to a focus on women whose paid work typifies what may be described as 'women's work'. A taken-for-granted feature of British employment patterns, 'women's work' involves its participants in restricted working hours, low pay, poor prospects and lowered status. They perform work of a feminine nature in a narrow range of occupations such as clerk, cleaner, caterer and carer. Looking to the literature on older women's lives, it is also clear that low lifetime earnings, and the consequent inability to make adequate financial preparation, has a profound impact on their future options and well-being. Furthermore, little is known of specifically female aspects of the transition to retirement. We therefore obtained the views of almost 100 women aged over 45 who were in part-time employment by asking them to discuss the relevance of their employment to their self-identity, their attitudes towards retirement and their views on PRE.

The findings prompted us to reconsider several elements of the literature that formed the study's background. First, although 'women's work' may appear to be somewhat disposable and insignificant, to the women concerned it was important, both financially and in terms of their self-identity as workers. Second, it was notable that they saw retirement through a framework built around notions of 'deserved leisure', reflecting a theoretical paradigm in which conventional, linear, masculine models of employment and retirement still dominate. However, they were also aware of changing gender and generational dimensions, suggesting to us the need to modify existing theory accordingly. Third, they viewed PRE as a useful resource and offered original ideas about its design and delivery that speak of a primarily strong and constructive approach to the prospect of becoming older women.

What follows is an appraisal of central points of correspondence and difference between the literature and the perspectives offered by a diverse sample of mid-life and older women engaged in 'women's work'. The chapter opens with an acccunt of the study methodology and concludes with reflections on the potential to incorporate the women's perspectives into theory and practice around the transition to retirement. The outcomes reveal ways in which myths, emerging from masculinised models of employment and retirement, are challenged by women's subjective evaluation of their worker identities and their determination to be actively involved in constructing their future identities as older women. In challenging these myths, the chapter exposes a need for new approaches to understanding women's ageing.

The study

There are two types of information to present in this section, and they may be termed the 'factual' and the 'abstract' sides of how the research took form. On the factual side, the first point to note is that the research was funded by the Pre-Retirement Association of Great Britain and Northern Ireland (PRA), a charitable organisation concerned, in this instance, with obtaining information on which to base appropriate help for women. Within the limitations of available resources, the research was designed to maximise the amount and utility of information on working women's requirements of PRE. It was therefore decided to approach women who were in part-time employment (as defined by their employer) and who were aged between 50 and 60 years. In the event, this proved to be too difficult because employers repeatedly informed us that they had recently restructured their workforce and no longer had many, if any, women who matched these criteria. After reducing the lower age limit to 45, removing the upper age limit and contacting a wide range of public and private sector employers in the West Midlands, six group interviews were arranged with a total of thirty-one women. The interviews were tape-recorded and usually lasted for at least 1 hour.

Second, after these interviews, questionnaires were designed to address the pertinent issues identified by the women. The questionnaires requested biographical information on age, marital status and occupational details, followed by a series of eleven, mainly open-ended, questions about the role of paid work in their life and their thoughts on retirement and PRE. The questionnaires were sent out to a further 225 women through the same employers (a council and a cleaning firm) and through one other borough council. In total, sixty-two (28%) questionnaires were returned. The total achieved sample in both phases therefore numbered ninety-three women. Key characteristics in terms of their age, occupations and marital status are displayed in Figures 2.1–2.3. In summary, although most of the women were married, a sizeable minority were not, and their occupational and age distributions also display considerable variation. The sample composition included some noteworthy diversity within this group of women in part-time work.

On the more abstract side, there are several points to note about our approach to the study. First, working with a body of literature which covers macrolevel changes in women's lives since the 1950s yet which often neglects the impact of these changes on their later lives, we were keen to add to the debate the voices of those whose experience and views we aimed to understand. Second, the study design was informed by principles emerging from feminist critiques of social research methods, which may be briefly summarised in this context as pointing to the need to recognise dynamics of power and social aspects of the relationship between researcher and researched. Power was initially placed with the women studied to the extent that their views were sought in interviews before designing a questionnaire for wider distribution. Most of these interviews were with groups of co-workers and took place on the premises of their employer. One advantage of this was that interviewees were in familiar company and surroundings. The corresponding disadvantage was that these were work-related, rather than informal or independent, locations.

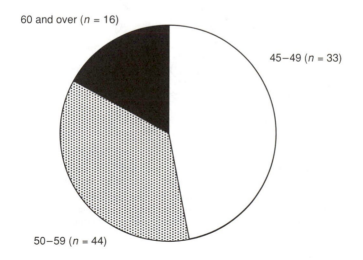

Figure 2.1 Age distribution.

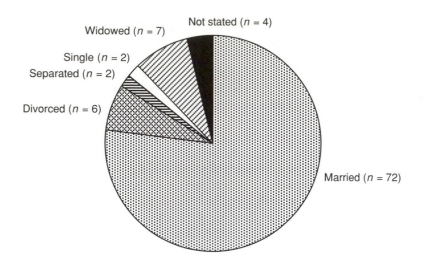

Figure 2.2 Marital status.

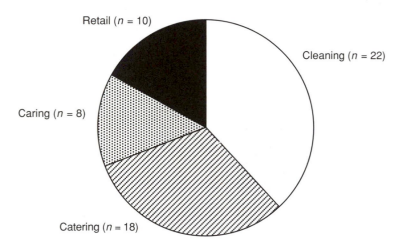

Figure 2.3 Occupational fields. Note: (a) Occupational information is drawn only from the questionnaire sample: fifty-eight of the sixty-two respondents provided this information. (b) Occupations within these fields include supervisory and management positions. (c) 'Caring' includes youth work and other social services. (d) 'Part-time' employment, as defined by employers, ranged from 8 to 39 hours per week.

Overall, therefore, the design and field work aimed, where possible, to recognise and to avoid pitfalls that might lead to what Jane Ribbens (1984) warns against in reducing women to manipulable data. Further to this, interpretation and analysis of the emerging data required a focus on offering an accurate picture of the women's perspectives. It would be rather too simplistic to overlook the fact that this process involved some reflection on appropriate ways to present anomalies between subjective and objective viewpoints on certain issues. However, it was precisely in the process of dealing with these anomalies that the research began to shed light on significant issues. For example, although the women recognised the objectively low value of 'women's work', they asserted its personal value, and whereas they often saw retirement as something for men (full-time continuous workers) many also aimed to approach their later life with optimism that it would entail similar benefits for them. It is also useful to note that, in the absence of the women's consensus over several issues, displaying diversity among a relatively small group of mature and older women in similar employment circumstances became a key aim of the analysis.

'Women's work'

In the second half of the twentieth century, one of the main changes in women's lives was the growth of their involvement in the labour market. Yet, as Jean Martin and Colin Roberts (1984) and Catherine Hakim (1993) assert, part-time employment was a major component of this growth. Contesting Hakim's (1998) argument that this is a matter of women's preference rather than a result of structural influence, Rosemary Crompton and Fiona Harris (1998:119) propose that:

> …women's employment behaviour is a reflection of the way in which women actively construct their work-life biographies in terms of the historically available opportunities and constraints.

To understand the interaction of individual choice and structural factors in shaping their perspectives on paid work, it is necessary to contextualise the employment situation of the women studied in relation to the opportunities and constraints operating during their working lives. The youngest women in the study would have entered working age in the early 1960s and the oldest in the mid-1940s. This places them within the cohorts for whom the post-war economic boom entailed new opportunities for employment, especially on a part-time basis in the expanding service sector. In parallel with this, social change enabled women to continue in employment after marriage and, increasingly, after the birth of their first child (Martin and Roberts, 1984; Audrey Hunt, 1988; Blackburn and Jarman, 1993). In short, these women were among those whose working lives were formed in a period of change that sets them apart from earlier generations of women. Similarly, they differ from later generations of women for whom full-time and more continuous patterns of employment have become more common. However, between the 1940s and the 1980s, and therefore across their working lives, the female part-time discontinuous pattern of employment in gender-stereotyped occupations became firmly established as an integral feature of the British labour market. By 1991, almost 5 million women (40% of those in employment) in Britain had part-time paid work (Department of Employment, 1992). This figure represents one-third of the total female part-time workforce in the European Community (EC) (Equal Opportunities Commission, 1992), offering a clear indication of its relevance to the British economy and thereby displaying the opportunities and constraints surrounding the women studied.

Age also plays a part in the likelihood of women taking part-time employment in terms of the individual working-life profile. The conventional post-war pattern of labour market participation involved exit during the family formation years, with returns likely to be on a part-time basis (Shirley Dex, 1987). Elias and Gregory (1994: 39) summarise the effects, as shown by their analysis of labour market data from 1975 to 1990:

> The typical woman in her twenties had full-time experience only; by her early thirties she was equally likely to have only full-time or some part-time experience; from her early forties she would typically have some part-time rather than only full-time experience.

By the late 1980s, over half of the women who were in employment as they approached retirement worked part time (Ann Harrop, 1990). This picture of women's employment is one that may be contested on the grounds that it overlooks the gains towards equality that were made in previous decades. The central point to note, however, is that those gains have not been universally enjoyed. Rubery and Fagan (1994) explain that there is increasing polarisation of women workers, with women part-timers tending to work in different occupations from both women and men in full-time employment. One consequence of this is that occupational segregation is reinforced, with part-time employment leading to women being more likely to remain working alongside other women and at lower hierarchical levels.

In relating the lived experience of the women studied to the overview presented above, perhaps the most telling finding was that the women displayed a strong sense of their position in a hierarchy of workers. At the top were men, who had full-time continuous work histories. At the bottom were earlier generations of women and young people, neither group being viewed as having had substantial involvement in the role of worker. The women themselves were therefore located in the middle. This typology was related to more than just employment though; it involved gender- and age-based perspectives on the extent to which the women thought the role of worker was an important feature of identity. Men were thought to view paid work as a far more important aspect of life than were women. However, the women in this study thought that both they and their female peers had a greater attachment to the worker role than women of earlier generations. Younger people were thought to have a less committed approach to employment, a view presented on the grounds that the women themselves felt that they had developed such commitment as part of the process of gaining maturity.

Further facets of the women's worker identities emerged in response to questions concerning the extent to which they valued their employment. Unanimously, they stated that paid work was an important part of their lives. It provided them with a social identity in addition to their familial one, social interaction with colleagues and clients, a sense of independence and a limited, but significant, source of income. Their own words offer clear expression of the importance of these factors:

> It might sound awful but it makes you a person in your own right doesn't it? I'm not just a wife and mother, I'm me, you know.
>
> > (Josie, catering worker in her mid-forties)

> It was nice to think somebody needs me again.
>
> > (Kath, social work assistant in her early fifties)

> I like having a job. I've always worked and I think it keeps me together actually. I do enjoy working.
>
> > (Sue, retail assistant in her mid-fifties)

Financial necessity was also brought to the fore on numerous occasions in the interviews, but more readily so in written replies to the questionnaires and especially by women who were not currently married. Widows appeared to have the greatest attachment to their worker role, often working beyond the age of 60 and hoping to continue for as long as possible, not least as an escape from isolation (an issue dealt with more fully by Pat Chambers in Chapter 8):

> I've lost my husband. This [job] takes me out of the house, does me good.
>
> (Laura, retail assistant in her early sixties)

However, the particular nature of 'women's work', which the women defined in accordance with the general view of it, was a prominent aspect of the women's understandings of the relative importance of work to men and women. Men were thought to have less choice in the matter of whether to take paid work and were thought to need employment for self-esteem and to fulfil their obligations as 'breadwinner'. In contrast, many said that women's relationship with employment was at a more humble level:

> Women can do little jobs…cleaning etc., which men wouldn't do.
>
> (Catherine, cleaner in her late fifties)

There was a slight difference in attitude among the younger women studied, who were more ready to indicate their disapproval of this gender distinction. As one commented:

> Women are prepared to take any work they can do if they need the money. Men tend to be too choosy.
>
> (Chris, clerk in her late forties)

Finally, it is noteworthy that although few of the jobs held by the women were considered to have intrinsic merits, there was hardly any mention of negative aspects of their employment. When complaints were voiced, they tended to focus on low pay, practical difficulties of managing both home and employment responsibilities, and problems with transport to work. In short, they reiterate the problems of 'juggling' responsibilities discussed by Judith Phillips in the next chapter.

To summarise, 'women's work' was a world that these women recognised as their own and spent part of their lives within. Although they accepted that it offered them little in the way of social status in comparison with 'men's work', they expressed a high level of attachment to simply being in employment. Without a partner, this attachment intensified. In relation to the background literature, it would therefore seem appropriate to conclude that these were women of their time, with an approach to employment that reflected the social, economic and individual circumstances in which they found themselves. Their decision to take up part-time employment was argued by many to be a matter of convenience, rather than free choice, as they believed that they were expected to combine domestic responsibilities with earning money. Their experiences and outlook therefore lent further support to the position expressed by Crompton and Harris (1998). Most of all, it must be stressed that, for the women concerned, 'women's work' was very important indeed.

Women don't retire...

...if they give up paid employment, they continue as a housewife.

(Mary, cleaner in her sixties)

The above comment reflects a popular view among the women. Mary's words also have a resonance beyond the direct meaning conveyed as they point to a theoretical framework that presents retirement in the context of traditional male, continuous, full-time employment patterns. They also echo research which shows that the majority of older non-working women, even up to the age of 74, would not describe themselves as retired (Laczko and Phillipson, 1991). In this section, we briefly outline conceptions of retirement, developed since the 1940s, before pointing to issues specific to the lives of older women for which PRE might help them prepare. The women's perspectives on their retirement, in terms of their expectations, hopes and fears, are then brought forward to compare understandings and to highlight levels of awareness of what the transition entails.

Early theories about retirement adopted the then dominant functionalist perspective on society, with writers of the 1940s and 1950s proposing that retirement was the end of an adult's economically and socially productive life and something which should be approached with a readiness to withdraw from society. The emphasis was therefore on disengagement and the significance of social roles, and men's transition to retirement was the central concern. A key change in theoretical work in the area was the introduction, in the 1980s, of the political economy perspective. Retirement became viewed as a political construction through which earlier social inequalities continued, and yet gender bias in the overall framework of thought was not eradicated (for example, Phillipson, 1982). More recently, it has also been suggested that life may be separated into four ages, with retirement (and/or early retirement) marking the onset of the 'third age'. Elsewhere, Miriam Bernard and Kathy Meade (1993a) and colleagues have discussed the shortcomings of established theory in relation to the transition to later life of women. To summarise, a central problem is that women's lives fit least readily into models that compartmentalise life stages. Instead, it is more useful to think in terms of interwoven life-course strands, employment being but one of these, thereby representing more fully the complexity of women's lives. In short, women such as those who participated in the study are in danger of being left out of, or misunderstood through, linear masculine models.

It is therefore useful to begin discussion of the women's perspectives on later life by returning to consider the implications of Mary's popular assertion that women 'don't retire'. One possibility is that the term 'retirement' has itself become laden with a gendered meaning. In addition, the continuation of domestic responsibilities to which Mary refers implies that unpaid 'women's work' also blurs the perceived boundary into later life. The last point was strongly evident, as the following quotations show:

> When a married couple retire the women seem to spend most of the time doing housework etc., whereas men *do* retire.
>
> (Helen, clerk in her early fifties)

> In many cases men still think of retirement as 'stopping' everything. Women know that the routine chores at least still have to be done.
>
> (Gill, clerk in her late forties)

Despite this difference, many of the married women in this study anticipated a renewal of their relationship with their husband once they had both relinquished paid work. Although they generally hoped for time to enjoy their leisure together, some also noted that adjustment would be required:

> A lot of women that I've talked to who've retired say [that the problem is] coping with their husband in retirement.
>
> (Josie, catering worker in her mid-forties)

There was also a recognition of women's greater longevity in their comments about the prospect of widowhood (issues which are discussed by Linda Machin and Pat Chambers in Chapters 7 and 8). As with many features of the women's expectations, fears of widowhood were expressed through reference to other couples:

> So many people we know who've retired, men at 65 women at 60, haven't even had a chance to enjoy their retirement.
>
> (Jane, retail assistant in her mid-fifties)

The widows were also the older women in this study, and their decision to remain in employment was closely associated with having lost their partner. As two retail assistants in their early sixties explained:

> We're both widows, so what is there for us at home?

When the women spoke of retirement in general terms, their fears included the prospect of living in poverty, isolation, boredom and, although few mentioned it, physical frailty and dependency. However, hopes were as likely to be expressed as fears. These centred on the possession of freedom and time, combining together into a comfortable liberty to enjoy travel, relaxation and socialising. It is important to note that most women tended to focus on either their hopes or their fears, and the polarity of views may be seen as an indication of a common reluctance to engage in unprompted thought about later life.

One of the more illuminating topics raised was that of likely differences between later life for these women and for those of their mothers' generation, and improvements were identified on many levels. First, earlier generations had sometimes been compelled to remain in employment through financial necessity. Greater affluence was therefore the source of a range of new options. Changes in the social position of women, and in attitudes toward ageing, were also noted. Key differences were summarised in a range of ways:

> My mother worked until she was 74. Now, since she lost Dad, she's just sitting in the house. [Work] kept her going.
>
> (Freda, catering worker in her late fifties)

> Hopefully, I shall have a more enlightened outlook on life and not take [ageing] to mean I cannot try something new. Not switch off and live in the past.
>
> (Clare, clerk in her late forties)

> They were really old before their time in those days…we're so lucky today.
>
> (Sheila, retail assistant in her early fifties)

In keeping with established theoretical frameworks, there was a tendency for later life to be understood by these women in terms of distinct stages. Loss of the worker role was something that most of the women did not look forward to, however much they might express optimism about the future. That, however, was feared far less than widowhood, which many determined to be a more important event than retirement, implicitly representing the onset of their old age. Most of all, there was a tendency to draw a clear line between the (desirable) early, active phase of later life and, as they saw it, the (dreaded) condition of eventual dependency.

To summarise, the women placed themselves in a hierarchy. At the top were men, who moved into a new world as retirees, free from their primary role in life and therefore liberated to do as they pleased. At the bottom, were earlier generations of women for whom the option to give up paid work may not have been available and for whom retirement was largely a process of withdrawal and a life of difficulty. The women in this study positioned themselves in the middle to the extent that they expected to have a later life similar to that of men, at least in terms of enjoying their leisure in comfort before widowhood and eventual dependency. Gender differences would prevail, however, in that they expected to have to continue to carry full responsibility for their unpaid work in the home. This, the women's work from which they could not retire, was resented but accepted as a feature of established norms.

Preparing for later life

Preceding sections display a rather particular set of conditions and attitudes that separate these women from others, both younger and older than themselves, and from men, suggesting perhaps that they have no role models to follow as they approach their later lives. They are, however, aware of what ageing may or must entail through witnessing the experiences of others. So, although their transition to retirement can be said to be characterised by both gender- and age-specific features, some of its aspects must be expected to mirror more general experiences of change. This raises a number of questions about how they are to prepare themselves for later life. One of the clearest messages that they wished to convey was that they had firm confidence in their ability to cope. Although this is explicitly a statement of optimistic resilience, it may also be viewed as an embodiment of an expectation of neglect or their resignation towards a perceived inevitability. The forms of help offered by pre-retirement education (PRE) are premised upon the view that it is not necessary to cope alone with the experiences accompanying the transition into later life. A brief account of its development, aims and approaches establishes a setting in which to place the women's views of their requirements.

PRE originated in the USA in the late 1940s and was introduced into Britain in the mid-1950s. Molly Heath (1976: 16–17, cited by Phillipson and Strang, 1983: 8) describes the intentions of an early British course. The aim was to help participants through the initial months of retirement,

> ...when anxiety, depression and introspection might do infinite harm, and to give them a boost, to give them all the practical, factual help they might require.

In contrast to the growing social gerontological basis of much of the American provision, PRE in Britain was less closely associated with a theoretical framework and, until the 1970s, both provision and course content were restricted. In keeping with role theory's emphasis on the significance of the loss of the worker role to men, the focus was on helping men in the final stages of their working lives to find ways to substitute new roles to cope with the impending loss (Phillipson and Strang, 1983). In 1961, Patrick Heron identified the six areas of focus for PRE as health, finance, housing, friendships, interests and personal philosophy of life (Kathy Meade and Joanna Walker, 1989: 180). More recently, the PRA has turned its attention to developing models to help a wider range of people with mid- and later life changes, and Meade and Walker (1989) have proposed that suitable provision for women would incorporate a fairly radical revision of traditional models.

The historical development of PRE, and its perceived social merit, cannot be disassociated from wider economic and social changes. In the context of an ageing population (Bernard and Meade, 1993a), a 'greying' workforce (Walker, 1993) and the increase in more flexible forms of employment, especially among women (Hutton, 1996), there are a number of issues to consider. For example, later life, when defined as the period following retirement, may well account for 20 years or more of an individual's life, stimulating greater need to make adequate preparation.

Demographic changes entail that a growing proportion of the workforce will be over the age of 45, indicating a possibility that employers may become more dependent on older staff, thereby potentially altering the way in which retirement is viewed. As women's participation in the labour market continues to increase, 'women's work' and associated demands for flexible working become more firmly embedded in the social structure, potentially reducing the extent to which individuals may predict and prepare for their future.

The majority of the women in this study were found to be ready to take up an offer of PRE, but the potential for practitioners to help them to prepare for the transition is dependent upon a range of factors. At the most practical level, there are issues of access. Most simply, the low status of 'women's work' may reduce the likelihood of employers offering such provisions. Approximately one-quarter of the women studied were employed by organisations that offered PRE to their staff, but this is more a function of sample selection than an indication of the level of provision. Further to this, while some of the participating employers made efforts to arrange a comfortable room for interviews and allowed staff to contribute during their working hours, others considered it appropriate for us to meet afterwards and in changing rooms. It would therefore seem necessary to consider a variety of routes outside the traditional connection through employers, perhaps including the women's suggested use of colleges and advice centres to facilitate contact.

It is important to note that there were different levels of interest in PRE among the women. Those most interested were currently single, relatively young and in higher level occupations. In relation to age, it would therefore seem that conventional approaches, timed to coincide with the latter phase of employment, might be less appropriate than a mid- and later life model of PRE. The occupational level disparity remains a difficult question to address. For example, higher level occupations are associated with higher earnings which, in turn, enable a more confident approach to financial planning. Additionally, women in such occupations may be more educationally confident than others and therefore more open to educational programmes. Bearing in mind such potential variations, an exploration of the women's requirements of PRE displays how content and mode of delivery might be subjected to the revisions proposed by Meade and Walker (1989).

Finances were the women's central area of interest. Alongside advice on how to prepare, through pensions, savings and investments, they wanted both preparatory and continuing help to be available with regard to claiming benefits and budgeting on a low income. There was general agreement that unless they began to prepare early there would be little possibility of making adequate financial arrangements. Some aspects of Heron's (1961) model of PRE were given relatively little attention by the women, with housing issues having low priority and health advice being rejected because of their absolute certainty about how to manage their own health needs. Friendships were mentioned in the context of taking steps to avoid social exclusion and isolation. However, as Dorothy Jerrome (1993) suggests, these were not generally considered to be a particularly significant component of successful adjustment to, and enjoyment of, later life. In contrast, Heron's 'personal philosophy of life' was identified by some women as a key factor to this end, with the development of positive attitudes towards ageing being expected to have an important influence on their behaviour and experience. This accords with the conclusions of Maxine Szinovacz (1982), drawn from her review of the experience of women in America. However, Szinovacz (1982) also states that women's preparation for later life must incorporate preparation for widowhood, and although the women in this study identified this as a major issue they did not include it as a subject for PRE to address.

The women's preferences for modes of PRE delivery display some of the ways in which the general or practical, and the more personal or sensitive, subjects may each be dealt with to greatest effect. The most important finding in this respect was that the women wanted to be active participants in the PRE process, rather than passive recipients of an educational programme delivered in a traditional teaching style. Group discussions were the favoured form of delivery, particularly in combination with expert advice. This mode would address their wish to gain assurance that their concerns were 'normal', along with providing opportunities to benefit from the experience of others. It would therefore be an ideal format for dealing with the financial, social and attitudinal aspects that they identified and might also be a way in which expertise, experiential or otherwise, could be introduced to raise other issues such as health and housing. Written or videoed material were favoured over lectures as a general method of delivery, and these could therefore be utilised to address the more intimate or feared issues of widowhood and the later stages of life.

Conclusion: reflections on theory and practice

The transition to retirement from 'women's work' is one in which women move from a feminised sphere of the labour market into a later life that has been theorised through what may be termed a masculinised framework. In other words, at the end of the twentieth century, the mature women in this study, who had followed a conventional pathway through employment, were approaching their later life carrying consequences that are little understood. Recent feminist interest in older women has exposed the need for gender-specific attention to be paid to many areas of later life. The study reported here provides evidence to support the development of new ways of addressing the transition into later life of a rather particular, yet in many senses gender typical, group of women. A review of the key findings prompts suggestions for fresh perspectives in gerontological theory and PRE practice.

First, this study shows that 'women's work' is vitally important to the women who perform it. This short sentence contains a host of meaning, not least an aim to dispel commonplace ideas that relegate it to a disposable, relatively worthless, if not risible, form of employment. Women who perform low-skilled, low-paid, low-status work on a part-time basis are engaged in a sizeable, well-established and flourishing area of the British labour market. Their position reflects the structural constraints and opportunities surrounding them, as Crompton and Harris (1998) argue, and as many of the women in the study indicated. Subjectively, the role of employee is of considerable importance, bringing into their lives an independent source of social identity and limited, but prized, financial strength.

Second, in the absence of paid work, the women expected, with reluctance, to have to continue with sole responsibility for domestic duties. This was but one of the ways in which the retiree role was identified as being highly gender specific. Their views on later life may be summarised as a mixture of hopes and fears; the former relating to an affluent, companionable period of leisure in the earlier years, the latter referring to a dread of widowhood, isolation and poverty. Partners were therefore a central component of the ways in which expectations were formed. Indeed, for those women who had already become widows, employment was a mainstay and they were reluctant to even consider the prospect of giving it up. The point to note here is that the expected meaning of retirement is crucially dependent on a woman's partnership status.

Third, there are a number of disparities between conventional models of PRE and women's requirements of preparatory help with the transition. Finance features largely in the women's interests, but they emphasised that assistance with this would be needed in mid-life more than at the close of their working lives. They also rejected the idea of being offered help to prepare for the health problems with which they are likely to have to contend in later life, and the area of housing, despite its significance, was a low priority. Although they were ready to cope alone with the changes to come, there was a very high level of readiness to accept help. The women therefore proposed innovative ideas to shape PRE to suit their circumstances. These included improving accessibility by taking PRE out of the workplace and into both colleges and video format; expanding the notion of 'expert' advice to include experiential expertise from recent retirees; and extending the period of contact with practitioners from an initial mid-life meeting through to ongoing advice centres to use beyond the transitionary phase. In short, their perspectives expand considerably on the basic model of PRE. It is notable that these ideas may not have been exposed if the women's insistence that they would cope, an almost unanimous assertion, had been accepted as the last word on their relationship with PRE. A fourth point to note is that a research methodology in which women's perspectives were centralised, and therefore reached towards, enabled the study to move participants into a position of constructing their own framework of service provision.

Implications for developments in the field of gerontological theory may be expressed as opportunities to remedy the relative neglect of women ensuing from linear, masculine models of employment, retirement and PRE. The first opportunity lies in dispelling underestimation of 'women's work', both paid and unpaid. This leads to the potential to rethink what it is to live without paid work as a prime determinant of identity, an experience that co-exists with their part-time employment and succeeds the point of retirement for the women studied. The increasing trend to flexible employment may also undermine the concept of retirement as a clearly fixed point of transition out of paid work for other groups of workers. Retirement may therefore be viewed as both a gendered and changing concept, at the point of transition and beyond. Finally, the study's methodology reveals an opportunity for theory to benefit from reflections on variations in the subjective meanings of employment and retirement.

To conclude, the women who participated in this study have experiences to carry into later life which encapsulate a key aspect of women's relationships with paid and unpaid work in the second half of the twentieth century. Their worker identities, although trivialised by myths, are of great value to the women themselves. As they discussed their future selves, they provided indications of the factors of influence that will shape the lives of the next generation of older women. One of their strongest messages was that they intended to ensure that they have a key part to play in the construction of their identities and lives as older women.

3 Working carers

Caring workers

Judith Phillips

Introduction

One of the most important sociodemographic trends of the twentieth century was the marked shift in 'women's work' and family commitments. Changes in fertility together with later marriage have enabled increasing numbers of women to enter the labour market and pursue careers alongside raising a family. As labour market changes increasingly require women in the workplace, and job flexibility enables them to take greater advantage of such opportunities, more women in mid-life will be found in paid work. Some will be tempted back into paid work after having a family, whereas others will have remained in work, supported by childcare arrangements. At the same time, these women are more likely to be involved in the care of an older adult.

Existing literature highlights the conflict which potentially arises between employment and caring as women attempt to balance the two roles. For many women, however, it is not just two roles which are in question, but a variety of different roles and aspects of life which need to be juggled: work, family, domestic and leisure time and as employees, partners, mothers, daughters and carers. Research on the 'sandwich generation' (Elaine Brody, 1990) has documented the problems in relation to women with both childcare and eldercare responsibilities, but there are a variety of other situations where care of an older adult is combined with other responsibilities, such as carework in a paid capacity. There has, to date, been little research in this area.

Indeed, my initial interest in this issue arose as a daughter and carer for older parents living at some distance from both home and employment bases. Working formerly as a social worker with older people in a professional capacity, and currently as a social work academic, raised expectations of self and others of my caring and work roles. Pressures around the inability to respond quickly in emergencies, difficulties in being in two places at one time, in different roles as worker, daughter and carer and the feelings of guilt and helplessness heightened my interest in how careworkers who had informal care responsibilities did in fact manage different roles in their everyday lives.

Thus, this chapter begins by broadly outlining the demographic changes taking place to make work–family transitions possible for women at mid-life. Attention then turns to a consideration of the importance of work to women's identity before moving on to look at the misconceptions and myths surrounding the lives of working carers. Drawing on this review of the existing literature, together with insights obtained from a focus group of women in mid-life, I argue against a 'static' role theory perspective and instead advocate a longitudinal life-course approach.

The demographics of care and employment

The burgeoning literature on informal care since 1988 reveals the various ways in which caring has been defined, depending on the type of care and hours devoted to unpaid caregiving (Gillian Parker, 1992). Likewise, what constitutes carework in a paid capacity is discussed by many authors (Clare Ungerson, 1997; Celia Davies, 1998). Clare Ungerson highlights the importance of considering both 'care' and 'work' together on the basis of contextual factors, both practical and conceptual. One of the contextual factors that has raised this issue high on the policy agenda in recent years has been the demographic imperative.

The demographics of care make it increasingly likely that women in mid-life have the 'structural potential' for caring (Anne Martin-Matthews and Carolyn Rosenthal, 1992) and will be entering the 'second wave of nurturing' (Gail Sheehy, 1995). The demographic shift over the last 30 years with increasing numbers of older people, particularly over 85 years of age, requiring care, together with the cutbacks in the available support from the public sector, has led to greater reliance on the family as providers of care to older people. Larger numbers of women, many of whom will be informal carers, are also entering the labour market; a trend which is expected to continue alongside the growth in occupations favourable to women, such as service industries (Heather Joshi, 1995). At the same time, the traditional male breadwinner model is breaking down (Rosemary Crompton, 1999). Consequently, there will be anticipated shortages in the supply of both female workers and informal carers. One way forward, it has been argued, would be to commodify informal care, putting it on a paid basis (Ungerson, 1997). Paid work and informal caregiving are therefore intimately related in this context.

The National Carers' Strategy (Her Majesty's Government, 1999) reveals that 41% of carers, predominantly women, are in mid-life (45–60 years of age). Two-thirds of working age carers (men and women) are also in paid employment of different kinds, equating to 2.7 million people combining work and informal care in Britain. Other studies carried out within specific workplaces, such as Avon Cosmetics, report that up to one-third of employees combine work and care for another adult (Kim Whatmore, 1990; Help the Aged, 1994; Ramsey, 1994). Furthermore, working carers' commitment to care, in terms of both time and task, is considerable. The National Carers' Survey (Whatmore, 1990) reports that 68% of the carers surveyed spent all their non-paid work time in caring. In a small survey of social work staff in Fife Regional Council, 11% said they spent virtually all their free time in caring (Ramsey, 1994). In a study of Avon Cosmetics, 3% of employees spent over 40 hours and 2% between 20 and 40 hours a week in caregiving (Help the Aged, 1994). Gender also continues to play a significant role. In many studies, women were primarily involved with personal care tasks such as feeding, bathing, getting people in and out of bed and helping them walk. They also participated in instrumental caregiving, although the differential between men and women in terms of financial help and companionship was much less. Greater time commitment to personal caring was evident for co-resident carers and those living or working in close proximity to the dependent adult (Judith Phillips, 1994; Ramsey, 1994). The Help the Aged (1994) study of Avon cosmetics found that 7% of employees were living with the older person, but 77% lived within half an hour's travelling distance. Time was primarily taken up with visiting older relatives, providing transport, companionship, shopping and help with general household tasks.

All workplace-based studies estimate that more people expect caregiving to increase in the future, and that it will affect their work in the years ahead. In specific workplaces, almost 60% of respondents from Avon cosmetics and Oxfordshire County Council, and 54% in the Fife study, anticipated new caring responsibilities in the next 5 years (Help the Aged, 1994; Ramsey, 1994).

Identity of working carers

Although notions of public (paid work) and private (domestic work) identity are seen as separate, they are often connected and in conflict (Rosamund Billington *et al.*, 1998). Work is bound up with an individual's sense of self-identity. Work, however, is highly gendered. Men's identity is still primarily constructed from their role in the workplace (Rosemary Crompton and Fiona Harris, 1998). National policies have reinforced this idea, for example by leaving women who choose to work to make their own arrangements for providing care. Despite increasing female employment and the loss of the traditional male 'breadwinner,' there has not yet been a significant shift in men's domestic roles, and women's income is still largely viewed as marginal to the household (Julia Brannen and Peter Moss, 1991). Several authors argue that such persistence of women's identification with domestic work is due to gender socialisation (Nancy Hooyman and Judith Gonyea, 1995; Crompton, 1999).

However, women's identity too is increasingly shaped by work. Yet women carry out different types of work from men and experience work differently. Being wives and carers is still crucial to the identities of many women. For working women, this raises potential contradictions and conflict in their self-identity between 'being' carers and 'doing' work (Billington *et al.*, 1998). In many cases, this domestic identity is transferred into paid work arenas, such as care work. This is often low paid and women are consequently locked into low-status roles and jobs (see Chapters 2 and 4). Rosemary Crompton (1999) found that where the male breadwinner earns more than his female partner household arrangements are more likely to be traditional. These arrangements are reinforced when the female is in a low-paid, low-status job. However, this also applies to high-status professions, such as the medical profession, where women attempting to juggle work and care responsibilities enter specialisms in which the hours of work can be manipulated. This resulted in reproducing conventional gender role divisions in the household (Crompton, 1999).

A post-modernist life-course perspective argues that a diversity of identities can coexist at different times in different places. The private domestic identity can be juggled with the public work identity. For example, in an in-depth qualitative study of sixteen carers looking after an older person with dementia, Diane Seddon (1998: 154) found that 'employment constituted an integral part of their identity'. For many, paid work was associated with independence and control over resources, as well as being recognised as something other than a carer. From a feminist perspective, it can be argued that the goal is to break down the dichotomy between work and home identities (Hooyman and Gonyea, 1995).

To explore experiences of caring in both informal and formal settings and to provide illustrative material for this chapter, a focus group of seven women was convened. Their names have been changed in the text to promote anonymity and confidentiality (Alice, Susan, Mia, Sarah, Rhian, Madeline and Val). All the women in the group were professionals, all were currently or previously involved in paid work involving older people and all had been, or were currently, informal carers. The group were all known to each other and met on one occasion for 2 hours to discuss the issues. In sharing their experiences, they contribute to the accumulating empirical evidence, which suggests that different identities can indeed be played out across the life-course. In so doing, this also enables us to challenge several of the myths and misconceptions still apparent in policy and practice.

Myths and misconceptions

Since the early 1980s, caregiving has been an issue which has received much attention in both research and feminist writing. But, despite such widespread consideration, myths still persist. The main sources of research and literature on this issue are US based, taking a logical positivist perspective. This in turn has influenced thinking in the British employment and caring literature. Together, this body of literature, while making important contributions to our understanding of paid work and informal care, also brings with it – and reinforces – several myths. In particular, we are presented with myths and misconceptions which highlight that:

- working carers are a homogeneous group;
- caregiving inevitably results in problems in employment;
- women substitute care for employment;
- it is a question of balancing different roles.

Working carers are a homogeneous group

The first myth places all carers in the same situation and facing similar problems. Most of the early research in the 1980s failed to disaggregate the different types of carer and often did not consider the situations they faced outside the caring relationship. The employment consequences of caring for an older person was one such ignored or marginalised area in early studies. From an employer's perspective, issues about caring and employment have mainly focused on child care. Adult care is different: often unpredictable, unpleasant, tinged with sadness and with much less recognition in the workplace. Structural and cultural issues around race, age and sexuality have been ignored in many studies. Yet, as family patterns change, different kinds of care exchange, for example between gay men and bisexual and lesbian women (Pringle, 1995), will need to be examined in relation to the workplace. Men too are increasingly engaging in caregiving of all kinds, challenging the notion that caregiving is all 'women's work' (Sara Arber and Jay Ginn, 1991; Fisher, 1994).

Caring situations are fluid and diverse, and large differentials exist in the ways that caring has an impact on employment, depending on a variety of factors. One important distinction is whether the carer is caring for a dependent outside or within the household. Pamela Doty and colleagues (1998) found that having the caregiver share the disabled person's home may reduce demand for paid help and reduce the need to cut back on paid working hours. Other research (Maria Evandrou, 1995) suggests the opposite – that co-residence precludes full-time work. Canadian research suggests that the location of home, workplace and elderly relative has a:

…discernible impact on levels of perceived stress and interference with work or family life, with travel time to work impinging primarily on the work side of the work–family balance, and travel time to elder primarily on the family side.

(Alun Joseph and Bonnie Hallman, 1996: 408)

They go on to argue that caregiving is a highly gendered spatial behaviour, with women and men caregivers providing assistance within very different time and space contexts. Women travel further (and longer) and do so more frequently to help older relatives with various tasks. This translates into women being more likely to adjust their 'time–space geographies' to provide assistance to their elderly relative and to meet other work and family obligations.

In our focus group, distance was certainly seen as contributing to women's differing experiences of work and care. Madeline looked after her widowed father and, living locally, provided the main practical support that he needed. She recalled:

My sister took no responsibility for what was happening as I lived nearest. But if I had not been there, it would have been different.

(Madeline)

Alice and Sarah also drew attention to the importance of distance:

My Dad lived an hour away. When he was well we used to go over as a family for recreation purposes. When he became ill it was a dilemma. He was near enough for me to do some things but far enough for me to be permanently exhausted. Yet, there was an expectation that I was near enough. In the care plan I was down as the one who did the shopping, yet it was difficult, as with work, I was exhausted and nearly crashed the car driving back home.

(Alice)

My brother lives 200 miles away, but when my parents moved they decided to be near us. It's the more psychological and emotional things that are difficult; My brother says 'ring me if I'm needed' – meanwhile, you carry the emotional stress rather than him because of the distance. He has emotional distance. He has to be needed before they ring him.

(Sarah)

As the last quote illustrates, other factors affecting the relationship between caring and participation in employment include the type of attention needed and the number of others who share caring tasks. As studies point out, it is the sole co-resident female carer who is most restricted in participating in the labour market. Men are less likely to be caring on their own and are much more likely to be in a supporting role to their partners (Arber and Ginn, 1991).

Similar differentials exist in relation to the intensity of caring. Eithne McLaughlin (1994) estimates that the crucial cut-off point is 20 hours of caregiving per week. Above this threshold, there is a decrease in the employment rate and a decrease in the proportion of carers working full time. The National Carers' Strategy, however, reports that 20% of working carers care for more than 20 hours per week.

Other studies point to the influence of class in the equation. Clare Ungerson (1987) found that women become 'career carers' when their husbands earned sufficient to support them; those on low or single incomes had no option but to combine work and care. Sara Arber and Jay Ginn (1993), in their analysis of the 1990 General Household Survey data, found that the middle classes were able to care 'at a distance,' being able to purchase care in the formal sector.

The nature of employment is also not homogeneous. Taken together, the range of possible work-life situations is enormous. Rosemary Crompton (1999) explores a range of possible earning (breadwinning) and care alternatives along a continuum ranging from the male breadwinner/female carer model, through dual earner/female part-time care, dual earner/state carer, dual earner/marketised carer to dual earner/dual carer. Each may have a different impact on work and care. In Britain, the dual earner/female part-time carer arrangement has emerged over the last two decades. Yet, in some employment practices, traditional gender relations (male breadwinner/female carer model) persist in the way work-life issues are conceptualised.

This section has highlighted the difficulties in describing a 'typical' working carer. Working carers are not homogeneous; different caregiving arrangements will have different impacts on a carer's employment.

Caregiving inevitably results in problems in employment

Recent studies taking a human resource perspective have concentrated on the negative effect that caregiving has on productivity (Help the Aged, 1994). Such negatives include losing concentration on the job, tiredness at work, having to take time off, arriving late and leaving early from work. Many working carers have to use work resources such as the telephone to arrange care services and hospital appointments. Taking time off work is reported by 40% of employees in both the Help the Aged studies compared with 15% of carers in the Fife study (Ramsey, 1994). Similar proportions are found in studies of medium-sized employers, such as the Anglia Harbours Trust NHS (Marion Graveling, 1989) and Rowntree Macintosh (Phillips, 1991).

On a personal level, such problems leave carers feeling guilty and worried about their job security. Feelings of dependency, and of not wanting to burden colleagues, leads to missed opportunities for promotion and restricted job opportunities. In our focus group, Mia, who was primary carer to her mother, who was suffering with multiple sclerosis, highlighted the temptations to relinquish her studies and social work career:

> This was a terrific pressure because the [paid] carer would leave at say 4 p.m. and I needed to be there shortly afterwards. If I was late on placement, or stuck on the M25, then I had to telephone mum's neighbours and let them know I would be late. I would stay with mum give her tea, chat, help with continence, shower, undress and help her to bed and read to her etc., then go home and start studying or spend some time with my partner. We had a bizarre existence and it was extremely stressful and pressurised.
>
> (Mia)

Sarah and Val expressed similar anxieties:

> As far as work was concerned I felt very guilty. I was always wondering what she [mother-in-law] was getting up to during the day when I wasn't there.
>
> (Val)

> Work wasn't a constant burden, but I felt resentful when I couldn't take time off. I found myself getting ill in the holidays – my problems seemed to fit around work.
>
> (Sarah)

Such descriptions reveal some of the less tangible and hidden problems that women experience when balancing work with caregiving, such as depression, emotional stress, anxiety, financial strain and the use of vacation time to care for others. Ways of coping with such difficulties include taking part-time work or changing jobs to cope with the problem (Help the Aged, 1994; Phillips, 1994), although none of the women in our focus group had done this. The most common reported effect, both in the focus group and in other research, is in adjusting work schedules to accommodate caring.

However, despite the difficulties experienced at work, there is little empirical evidence that productivity is adversely affected. It can also be argued that productivity is a male construct based on the norms of male capitalist success (Toni Calasanti, 1999). Indeed, feminist gerontologists would advocate that terms such as 'productivity' be reconstituted to begin with the work of women and encompass their unpaid labour (Ruth Ray, 1996; Calasanti, 1999). Furthermore, and by way of contrast, positive effects of caring and working can be found in other studies. A survey of Open University (1995) staff revealed that 29% found it rewarding and 38% said it helped them put other aspects of life into perspective. From an employer's point of view, working carers were more responsible, sympathetic and responsive. As Isabel Rossi (1995: 62) notes, 'Managing the dual role may make employees more organised and committed and dedicated to their work.'

As illustrated by our focus group, there are difficulties faced by women in the workplace and adjustments are made to cope with such pressures, but the myth that productivity is severely affected is not borne out by wider empirical research whereas the positives of the presence of carers in the workplace has not always been highlighted.

Women are substituting care for employment

Over the last decade, there has been a decrease in male participation in the labour force, with a concomitant increase in women's, albeit mainly part time, employment. For example, 22% of women under the age of 60 worked part time in 1991 compared with only 1% of men under the age of 65 (Department of Employment, 1992). One logical conclusion of this is that women are switching their roles from being the primary carers of older people to being employees in the workplace. However, the movement of women into such employment has not in fact reduced their availability for care, and many have in fact increased their commitments alongside increasing employment (Wolf and Beth Soldo, 1994; Doty *et al.*, 1998). Pamela Doty *et al.* (1998) and Stohs (1994) both argue that the 'ethic of care' still strongly influences women's behaviour, more so than the 'ethic of equity'. Phyllis Moen and colleagues (1994) found clear evidence of this in their study of 293 women from four birth cohorts. They found that women were equally likely to become caregivers whether or not they were employed.

Eliza Pavalko and Julie Artis (1997), in their research into employment and caregiving in late mid-life, conclude that the relationship is unidirectional, with women reducing paid working hours to meet caregiving demands. Whereas a compromise between work and care has existed for women, for men it is seen more in conflict (Janet Finch and Jennifer Mason, 1993; Joshi, 1995), with employment trends falling as caregiving increases. Men's lack of access to part-time work may have an influence on these patterns (Gillian Parker and Dot Lawton, 1990). Alternatively, men may not want part-time work as it affects their promotion and career advancement as well as identity. There is also evidence to suggest that men in conventional jobs often have to rely on the goodwill of their employer, rather than adapt their work around caregiving duties (Julia Twigg and Karl Atkin, 1994).

As Mia, who had cared for her mother with a long-term disability, comments:

> The possibility of giving up was very much on my mind as I didn't know how I could continue to cope with no end in sight and, also, my family, especially my grandfather, was very critical of me trying to continue with my career. He saw this as a selfish act and was very angry with me for a time. Inevitably, he was worried for his daughter but clearly saw it as my role. The possibility of my brother giving up work for example would never have entered his head, and he didn't criticise him either.
>
> (Mia)

However, for Mia, 'I worked so hard to get there I felt terrified to give up in case I never found a way back'.

Women's employment is not only affected during the caregiving period but there are also long-term economic disadvantages for the carer. Maria Evandrou and David Winter (1992) found evidence of depressed wage rates. Working carers' average earnings are below those of non-carers, and this differential is most marked for sole carers. It is not surprising therefore that single daughters are particularly reluctant to give up work (Jane Lewis and Barbara Meredith, 1988). Heather Joshi (1995) estimates that a woman carer who otherwise worked full time would forego earnings of £75,000 over 5 years of caregiving, as well as seeing a final pension reduced by £1,250 per annum. Consequently, not only are current incomes affected but future pension entitlements are also disrupted (Brannen *et al.*, 1994).

Thus, the picture emerging from research is one of women attempting to take on roles both as carers and employees, rather than the myth that they are choosing to relinquish care in preference for employment.

It is a question of balancing different roles

There is excessive attention, particularly in the psychological literature, on stress, burden and role overload among carers. Role theory, with its focus on role stress, has been the guiding concept. Such theory suggests that competing and conflicting demands of care and work will result in role strain, and there will be friction among work, care, domestic life, leisure and other social roles (Goode, 1960; Karen Fredriksen and Andrew

Scharlach, 1997; Mary Stephens and Aloen Townsend, 1997). When this strain becomes excessive, it leads to role overload (Barbara Murphy *et al.*, 1997), which is highest for those women in paid employment with childcare responsibilities (Andrew Scharlach and Sandra Boyd, 1989). Intermediary factors such as level of support within the household and the relationship between the carer and care receiver (Lawrence *et al.*, 1998) have been influential in relieving stress, as Mo Ray discusses in Chapter 9. Additionally, the accessibility and availability of formal support has consequences for perceived stress. This has in itself been criticised by feminist writers as it has led women into a spiral of dependency – informal carers, relying on female volunteers or other women in low-paid caring roles (Gillian Dalley, 1996).

The compensation model and the segmentation model offer some way towards a more positive framework (Zedeck and Mosier, 1990). The compensation model suggests that what people lose through their caregiving role, for example friends, they can make up in the workplace. The segmentation model separates out work and care in terms of time, space and function and argues that paid work can offer relief from certain aspects of caregiving. Several women in the focus group referred to the advantages of having work to act as a relief from caring at home. Val, at 45, was caring for her mother-in-law, who lived locally. She worked as a child psychologist: 'I didn't want to think about giving up work as my whole world would close down. I could actually *think* at work'. Sarah reiterated this: 'It was helpful having friends and colleagues at work going through similar things. It was very helpful and compensated for the work pressures.' Other studies also illustrate the advantages of employment for carers. Mary Gilhooly and Calum Redpath (1984) found that part-time work constituted an emotional outlet for female carers. For others:

> At times it was a great pressure to be under and I felt guilty about my feelings, selfish perhaps? However, being a home carer I feel more able to help people who are having a tough time caring for someone and can assure them that most people feel guilty and upset at times.
>
> (Ramsey, 1994: 8)

In particular, women in our focus group challenged traditional role theory as simply the 'balancing' of different roles and felt that 'juggling' was a much more appropriate term. Balance implies a certain degree of control, but they felt that the true situation was more akin to '*a roller-coaster of care*', being unpredictable, at times uncontrollable, chaotic and stressful, not a calm conscious balancing of roles. Alice and Rhian described it in these ways:

What might have appeared as a balancing act to everyone else wasn't how I saw it – I did everything. I was always the one contacted first if anything went wrong. It was heavily weighted in one direction. When I went to full-time work it felt more of a balance but I never consciously thought I'm going to balance – I thought I could do it all.

(Alice)

Being a long way away it felt like juggling rather than balancing – some balls got too heavy and then the problems started.

(Rhian)

Whether women are balancing or juggling, they seem to want increasingly to 'do it all' – in Rosemary Crompton's term, to 'maximise' – to be successful in the public sphere of paid employment and in domestic relationships as well (Crompton, 1999). Moreover, in recent years, a number of studies have further disputed role theory, finding little evidence for either role strain or role enhancement (Margaret Penning, 1998). The image of 'being caught in the middle' between competing commitments is also not a typical experience (Rosenthal *et al.*, 1996). Besides, role theory is individualistic and is not family based: it does not take into account the care receiver or any level of interdependence and reciprocity within the family (Rosalie Young and Eva Kahana, 1989).

Despite its predominantly US empirical base, role theory continues to be used to explore the negative effect of caring on work performance in workplace-based studies. Such studies attempting to measure burden and stress, however, are overly simplistic, cross-sectional and unidimensional, assuming a simple cause-and-effect relationship without including the subjective interpretations of working carers. Alternative conceptual frameworks building on role theory (Margaret Neal *et al.*, 1993), or using a transactional model where stress and burden are not necessarily viewed negatively by the carer (Nolan *et al.*, 1996), are increasingly influencing approaches to work and care. As yet though, this has failed to influence the way in which interventions are shaped.

In sum, role theory, with its psychological basis, has focused on women's weaknesses, placing the problem and solution in the control of individual women. A more useful approach can place intervention at the societal level, with caregiving viewed in its socioeconomic and political context. Exploring the meaning of care and work within the family, of how negotiations within the family are conducted and the impact of care on employment, and employment on family relationships, may also be a more fruitful way to proceed.

The myths and misconceptions discussed above are further illustrated and tested in the remainder of this chapter by looking at women who combine care in both informal and formal spheres and, in many cases, provide care over long periods of time.

The experience of paid and unpaid caring

Although these two spheres of care can be linked conceptually, there is still a dearth of empirical evidence to highlight the difficulties and rewards faced by carers who carry out both roles simultaneously. Celia Bevan and Susan Gattuso (1998), in their research based on focus groups of mid-life women, identify three models, which are discussed below. Drawing on our focus group discussion, a fourth model is added, highlighting how careworkers and professionals in social care cope with juggling two caregiving jobs. The first model (Bevan and Gattuso, 1998) illustrates how *maternal models dominate caring practices*, with beneficial and deleterious consequences for staff and consumers. Bevan and Gattuso (1998) argue that, because training is lacking, workers draw on their personal experiences of relationships with female relatives, predominantly their mothers. Replicating domestic situations is an extension of their traditional role compared with men who see work as their primary role.

Comments by our focus group also illustrated this:

> I think its very much a cohort thing. My mother worked so there was less expectation that I stayed at home and cared. It was the same when I had a child – there was an expectation that I would go back to work as soon as possible.

(Alice)

> One of our [focus] group discussed how her personal experiences of caring for her daughter and grandchild influenced her practice as a social work manager. I also had a fresh outlook and sensitivity to some childcare decisions at work.

(Susan)

However, practices such as taking on a maternal model in formal settings are shaped by the male view of work. In professional care too, the metaphors of masculinity have shaped work patterns and roles. Masculine representations such as individuality, self-reliance, formality and distance have translated into bureaucracies as 'being professional,' where emotion has no part to play. Emotional work is seen as 'women's work'.

In their second model, Bevan and Gattuso (1998) argue that *organisational culture conflicts with caring ideologies* and that there is conflict between being a professional and being a daughter. This was also highlighted by our focus group. Mia observes that:

> The hardest thing was being treated and viewed as a 'bad person' because I would not give up and because I was trying to juggle work and care. I could not get it right all the time. At times, I was accused of neglecting mum and did feel that I was not doing a good job. Others were critical of 'strangers' looking after her when it should have been me. I responded to this by believing they were half right – I was a bad woman for not caring and a bad daughter for not giving things up.

Mia's experience adds weight to studies such as those by Twigg and Atkin (1994), who argue that women tend to internalise tensions that arise in both roles. Such difficulties were present for professional social workers who had been trained to work with older people, as well as for care assistants who had not received any training.

Bevan and Guttuso (1998) go on to suggest that professional tasks cannot be ignored, but there needs to be a boundary to keep control – 'boundaries of the professional carer'. Keeping a professional face on the job implies a 'distance' between the carer and the user of their services. Julia Twigg (1999) describes how the use of gloves act as a symbol to enable professionals to keep their distance and act as a mark of professionalism. The move from social work to care management, with its emphasis on form filling and checklists, may also be an attempt to create distance from users, often in very disturbing and traumatic circumstances. Within the organisation, however, using Arlie Hochschild's (1983) concept of 'emotional labour', feelings of anxiety are manipulated to do the job of creating an environment of care. It is seen as unprofessional to display personal feelings to users, and accusations of 'overidentifying' with them can have severe disciplinary results. This difficulty was summed up by Sarah, who said:

> You have to admit you can't cope before you get support, yet you feel you should be coping.

Organisations, even those operating in the social care field, can however operate with a veneer of support, as in Alice's and Mia's experiences:

> College, in my view, were not very understanding about my commitments. In truth I did not ask them for support but when my mum died, I did feel hurt by their approach. It felt superficially supportive but cost them little. For example, they suggested I could 'take all the time I needed' – but this meant no longer than two weeks.

My college professor also said he would 'sort out' missing my examination and that I was not to give it a thought. On my return to college the first thing I had to face was resitting the exam at very short notice.

(Mia)

It's different long term to short term. At an informal level it was OK but if it had gone on longer I wonder how long the institution would have waited. Would I have been given permission by my colleagues?... There aren't any systems to support the juggling. You feel there is a right and a wrong way and a strong moral stance underlying all of this. There are dilemmas and complexities which you can't predict or plan for. You can't control it – it is like a roller coaster of care.

(Alice)

Finally, Celia Bevan and Susan Gattuso (1998) argue that *professional–personal boundaries* reflect the blurring of the public and the private in women's lives. Informal caregivers can lose a sense of self and become engulfed in the caring role (Twigg and Atkin, 1994) and this may have spillover effects in a professional role. Conversely, it has been argued (Davies, 1998) that careworkers take on an unacknowledged therapeutic role as they develop close relationships, which can be rewarding (Helen Jenkins and Chris Allen, 1998).

What is often seen as a distinction, but which has theoretically bound the two spheres together, is the concentration on the emotional intensity of the work. It is in this sense that the boundaries between professional and personal merge, as Sarah explained from her mother's experience following bereavement:

After my father died a nurse [Macmillan] came back to see my mum and talked about her husband who had dementia. My mum understood her problems and is still in contact. I'm not sure how clear the boundaries are as a professional carer, particularly if you are going through similar things. If a professional can't talk about their own role it seems difficult to give that emotional support. In the hospice movement they do get emotional support in their work role – it's part of their approach.

The experiences of our focus group participants suggest that it is possible to add a fourth dimension or model based on *knowledge and expectations* arising from a 'professional' role. Tensions can arise from expectations of the professional carer in informal care situations. Such expectations revolve around taking on the primary caregiving role, being knowledgeable about and understanding the situation and being able to cope with everything that is presented in the arena of 'care'. The following comments illustrate this:

> There was always an expectation that you could do more.
>
> (Val)

> As a social worker you should know about all these things such as benefits.
>
> (Rhian)

> I felt dreadful, even the day of his funeral, I saw the expectations on me and I couldn't fulfil the good daughter role. I don't know what they expected me to do other than what I had done, but you can never do enough. It's difficult as you didn't want to pull more clout than you deserve.
>
> (Alice)

The above statement from Alice highlights the difficulties of holding 'insider' knowledge, particularly when 'things went wrong.' However, there were advantages of being in this position, particularly when it came to negotiating your way through the system and talking to other professionals: 'I would know all the right questions to ask' (Madeline). Furthermore, careworkers and professionals in social care were often selected as the natural carer in the family and seen as the 'expert' because of working in that situation:

> My husband [who is a social work manager] would do all the phone calls. My Dad felt it odd – people would talk to me and I would know the right questions to ask. Geriatricians would talk to us. I carried clout as a social worker. It was frustrating when things went wrong. If you weren't in that role you wouldn't know they had gone wrong. There is also a danger that you collude with the professionals as you can see it from their point of view.
>
> (Alice)

Our focus group, however, reinforced the importance of hanging on to the personal rather than the professional role in their relationships with older parents:

> When my father went into hospital I became the daughter again. I was always his daughter and he as my father always supported me.
>
> (Alice)

Discussion: developing a life-course perspective

This chapter has demonstrated that most empirical studies use a cross-sectional approach while existing literature, drawn primarily from a human resources perspective, emphasises the psychological burdens in the dual roles of employee and carer. Women, throughout their lives, juggle different roles at different times, whether it is in response to child care, work, adult care or domestic life in general. Thus, transitions in mid-life, whether in relation to work and caring, in a paid or unpaid capacity, need to be seen within a life-course perspective.

Caring is often a long-term experience, particularly if the carer is involved in child care before caring for an older adult. In 1998, the Office of National Statistics found that 25% of carers reported having cared for someone for 5–9 years, and a further one-quarter had been looking after the person they cared for at least 10 years (Her Majesty's Government, 1999). Participation in the labour market can, therefore, be affected for long periods of time, with consequent impact on income and earnings.

There is also evidence to confirm that the effects of the intersection of work and care extend well beyond the end of the caregiving period or carework career, and will have an effect on the carer's own experiences in old age. The Office of Population Censuses and Surveys (OPCS) retirement survey (Janet Askham *et al.*, 1992) of third-age carers found that they had spent a smaller proportion of their adult life in employment than non-carers and, in many cases, had taken early retirement. Other studies found such carers spending a longer time in the workforce after state pension age than non-carers (Buck *et al.*, 1994; Tinker, 1994).

Deborah Merrill (1997) in her book on *Caring for Elderly Parents* draws our attention to three different axes along which a longitudinal perspective can be applied – the spatial, transactional and temporal. Experiences in one sphere, professional or personal (spatial), will be translated and adapted in responding to caregiving and career transitions in mid-life. Changes in work, family and health careers will all have an effect on each other. Merrill suggests that the extension of the caregiver role into professional carework indicates a predilection for lifetime involvement in caring. Carers may also enter formal care settings after relinquishing informal care roles.

A longitudinal life-course perspective also includes a transactional element incorporating the care receiver. Caring for an older person is shaped by previous relationships with them (Gunhild Hagestad and Bernice Neugarten, 1985). Experiences of women carers, whether they are in an informal or formal situation, are not shaped because they are women or because they are in paid or unpaid work, but because of the intersection of the two. Their experiences are shaped by what has gone before this current intersection. Also, a life-course perspective not only emphasises the 'interrelatedness of careers or role trajectories across the life course' (Merrill, 1997: 17) but also the temporal nature of caregiving. A current response is likely to be shaped by earlier experiences (temporal). Similarly, caring is not a static process; it can be sporadic or continuing and there is a need to monitor different periods of caregiving within a life-course perspective. In our focus group, for example, there was acknowledgement that similar situations were experienced by all women in the group earlier in their lives and careers, when work and care had crossed in relation to child care.

Balancing the roles of employee and carer has been the major focus of the research literature on work and care in the UK since 1980. This chapter has highlighted that several misconceptions have been founded on this approach, namely that carers are all the same, caregiving has negative effects on employment and that the stress of balancing the two roles is often so great that women abandon work. A more recent body of literature, empirically grounded and from feminist perspectives, illustrates that the initial reporting of the working carer's situation is too simplistic and purely negative, based on the conflict in women's identities between their private and public lives. In developing this issue further, we now need to take a broader longitudinal view of both work and care roles if we are to understand more fully what the experiences and implications are for women who are working carers and caring workers.

4 Our ageing selves

Reflections on growing older

Miriam Bernard and Val Harding Davies

Introduction

There are a number of well-rehearsed social and demographic reasons why a consideration of women and ageing – with a focus on the attitudes of mid-life women – is warranted and timely at this point. Briefly, we ourselves, and the societies we live in, are clearly ageing. Later life is now dominated by women and will continue to be so for the foreseeable future (Sara Arber and Jay Ginn, 1991, 1995; Miriam Bernard and Kathy Meade, 1993a; Moyra Sidell 1995). Furthermore, many of the so-called 'caring professions' are mainly the preserve of women – and women who, in all likelihood, will increasingly be caring for older women. 'Professional women carers', who are themselves ageing, also form an integral part of what Caroll Estes (1979) has termed 'the aging enterprise'. In other words, nurses, social workers and other caring professionals are part and parcel of the 'industry' which has grown up around ageing, and those of us who work in and alongside this 'industry' must recognise that we have professional and vested interests in it (Bernard, 1998).

Our own professional and vested interests in this topic have their origins in a number of interrelated sources. As two women in mid-life ourselves, we have worked with, taught and conducted research about aspects of ageing for women for many years. As teachers, we have been closely involved in running part-time postgraduate and post-qualifying courses in gerontology and counselling, which, by their very nature, attract large numbers of mid-life professional women (for example nurses, social workers, doctors and educators). As practitioners, we were also conscious that, in various guises, ageing seemed to be an issue for many of the women with whom we came into contact through our work in counselling and in the voluntary sector. In the early/mid-1990s, we became increasingly aware that although we were teaching about ageing and about counselling skills and techniques we very rarely examined these issues directly in relation either to our own lives or to the lives of our predominantly female students. In addition to writing and researching about ageing for women (Bernard and Meade, 1993a), one practical way that we began to address this was to offer optional annual workshops for female students undertaking the range of Masters programmes offered in the Department of Applied Social Studies at Keele University (in gerontology, social work and counselling). The workshop was entitled 'Our Ageing Selves', and attracted between twenty and twenty-five women each time it was run over a 3-year period.

With this as a background, the current chapter examines what mid-life women think and feel about growing older. First, we explore the available literature about women and ageing, alongside a consideration of the importance of paid, 'caring', professional work to women's identities. In so doing, we show how (as in Chapters 3 and 5 by Judith Phillips and Gillian Granville respectively) women in these years are engaged in a juggling act among work, self and family/domestic roles. Second, drawing on the results of a small empirical study, we examine the attitudes of female nurses to their own ageing and then go on to amplify the key themes through illustrative vignettes drawn from counselling practice. This empirical work and practice shows the complex mix of both expectations and fears that mid-life professional women have about ageing, and shows how difficult it is when confronted with the reality of some of these fears to construct and maintain a clear sense of one's own identity in the face of often overwhelming societal and familial pressures. Finally in this chapter, we reflect on ways in which we might usefully respond to these issues; it is our contention that until we, as mid-life women, fully explore and understand our own attitudes to ageing and old age, we will not be able to work in ways which are truly beneficial and empowering for the older women that we come into contact with in our professional capacities (Bernard, 1998).

Exploring the existing literature

As demonstrated elsewhere (Bernard 1998), a search of the academic literature around these issues is instructive in that it reveals substantive bodies of work on, for example, attitudes, older people and, even now, older women, as well as some literature on professional attitudes towards older people. However, we also find that there is very little work indeed which specifically examines the attitudes of older people themselves to a variety of practical and policy issues (Annette Boaz *et al.*, 1999). Furthermore, although the 'coincidence of age and gender' in the literature is to be welcomed (Dianne Gibson, 1996: 433), one key area in which we still lack data concerns the roles that gender and age play in terms of our own attitudes towards ageing. This dearth of research and writing in itself tells us a great deal about the invisibility of such issues. It also suggests to us that there is a widespread reluctance to even begin to ask the difficult questions about what ageing is like for us as mid-life professional women, let alone search for any answers.

Women and work: ageing and identity

Many authors have explored the ways in which gender operates in the workplace, highlighting, for example, the impact of the 'glass ceiling', of discriminatory employment practices and of gendered organisational cultures (see, for example, Catherine Itzin and Carole Newman, 1995; Catherine Hakim, 1996; Sylvia Walby, 1997; Rosemary Crompton, 1997, 1999). Importantly, this growing body of literature shows that women's identities are no longer simply associated with the traditional roles of wives and mothers, but that paid work and the social and psychological rewards it brings have their part to play in the ongoing development of women's identities (see also Chapters 2 and 3). However, in certain occupations, the continuing importance attached to the nurturing and caring skills that we still associate with being a woman have become institutionalised and are often a requirement of many of the jobs that women do in the paid labour market (Lisa Adkins and Celia Lury, 1992). This is clearly the case in nursing, where, as Celia Davies (1995) shows, our notions about what constitutes nursing are intimately bound up with ideas of what it is like to be a woman. Nursing goes to the heart of our identities as women, and is closely linked to the ways in which women's identities are connected with mothering and caring (Steph Lawler, 1996). Davies also goes on to demonstrate how difficult it is to completely divorce one's professional persona from one's view of oneself – even if one has been professionally trained to take account of perspectives which emphasise gender, age and race dimensions.

There are analogous debates and discussions among some of the other caring professions, particularly social work and counselling. Catherine Rees (1991), for example, in a study of social workers, old women and female carers, discovered that much of what passes for social work theory and practice does not contain a gender perspective, nor is it particularly sensitive to the problems which older women might encounter. This view is endorsed by Beverley Hughes and Melody Mtezuka (1992) in their examination of social work and old women. They lament the fact that texts which have attempted to develop alternative or radical practice have rarely, if ever, applied their thinking to work with older people or older women. In a similar vein, work from a counselling perspective looks at issues such as countertransference in therapeutic work with older people. This examines the ways in which a therapist's own emotional reactions to a patient or client (which might be based on past relationships, on ageist stereotyping or on other unresolved or ambiguous attitudes) might adversely influence the process of therapy. By acknowledging that such countertransference is a possibility, it is suggested that this provides opportunities for the helping person to examine his or her own reactions to issues such as ageing and death and, by so doing, to become a more competent helper (Greene, 1986; Genevay and Katz, 1990; Siegel, 1990). Again though, this kind of research tends to be generalised to the extent that it is often about professional attitudes towards older people, rather than specifically about mid-life female professionals' responses to older women or to their own ageing.

For further insights into women's experiences of ageing, it helps to turn to writing around the use of masquerade. Here, we can note in particular the contribution of feminist writers such as Ephrat Tseelon (1995), who articulates what she terms the masque of femininity in which, at one and the same time, one is able to present an exterior (or professional?) self to others while attempting to preserve a coherent, internal and personal sense of self. With respect to older women, the writings of Sarah Matthews (1979) and, more recently, of Kathleen Woodward (1991) show some of the ways in which older women actively use masquerade as a way of presenting a particular self or selves to others. This kind of strategy has also sometimes been referred to, and examined in the literature, as 'passing' or pretending to be younger than one really is (Barbara MacDonald and Cynthia Rich, 1984). Also, as Justine Coupland and her colleagues (1991) have shown, women of differing ages will in fact use differing strategies according to the context within which they find themselves – presenting oneself in a particular way to one's peers, but differently to younger women. Essentially, what this amounts to is a denial of ageing, but a denial which, in a culture and a society which systematically devalues, marginalises and discriminates against older people in general and older women in particular, is eminently understandable. Indeed, Simon Biggs (1999a: 82) cogently argues this point in his exposition of the second half of life:

> An inhospitable social climate has made the deployment of protective identities an effective strategy and point of resistance against such predations of the self and also a means of ensuring continued self-development... Masque, as an interaction of appearance and depth, has been made a necessity by changed life priorities that do not fit well with the age-ascriptions of the dominant culture; self-development by subterfuge against the ground of inhospitable constructions of age.

Some of the ideas sketched out above provide clues for helping us to understand what lies behind the findings of the only two specific pieces of

British empirical research to have focused on the interactions among women as professional carers, the older women they care for and the possible impacts that these have on their own identities and attitudes towards ageing.

Ageing women and older women

The first study to draw attention to this was carried out by Helen Evers (1981). She undertook a non-participant observation study of nurses and patients in eight geriatric wards of different hospitals. Her research showed that the nurses – who were themselves predominantly women – responded quite differently according to whether their patients were male or female (of the eighty-six patients observed, sixty-two were women). She found that women patients were far more likely to be depersonalised; the nurses knew a lot less about them than they did about their male patients; they were cared for in quite different ways; and they tended to be labelled as more 'difficult' than the men. The elderly women were identified as falling into three distinct stereotypes: the 'dear old Gran', the 'poor old Nellie' and the 'awkward Alice' types.

Evers (1981) shows how 'dear old Gran' types were popular, usually mentally alert and although sometimes physically frail were able to engage in animated and positive conversations with nurses. They were also notable for the fact that they never complained or criticised but 'fitted in' to the routines and practice on the wards and 'made the best of it'. Evers suggests that these women had surrendered their autonomy to the nurse, a similar strategy to that found in more recent, but similar, work conducted by Joanna Latimer (1997). 'Poor old Nellies', on the other hand, were more common and were often incontinent and fairly or heavily dependent on the nurses for many activities of daily living. The nurses tended to regard these women as 'unfortunate, helpless children', and any interaction was usually initiated by the nurse. If the women themselves requested attention, they would often be ignored by the nurses. Evers's third group, the 'awkward Alices', although in a minority, were mentally alert, articulate and assertive women. They exhibited a range of dependencies and, although capable of expressing gratitude to the nurses, they were also sometimes critical of nurses' attitudes and work practices. They came to be seen by the nurses as 'difficult patients' and, once labelled as such, it was very hard to shake off this label even if their behaviour changed. The nurses adopted various strategies to 'control' these women, including avoiding them, putting them on side wards, ignoring requests by always being preoccupied with other things, publicly rebuking the individual and leaving them until last.

Evers (1981) makes a number of suggestions about the possible reasons for these observed professional attitudes and behaviours: reasons which relate both to issues about identity and masquerade and to aspects of gendered ageism. First, she suggests that, in line with traditional roles and identities, female nurses find it less problematic to look after older men than older women for the simple reason that this is more closely related to what many of them do anyway. In other words, she too is arguing that nursing of this kind is an extension of women's 'natural' caring roles within the family. Second, this is further reinforced by the men also being 'in role' and being much more accepting of being looked after. In this instance, being a patient is an extension of men's conventional relationships to women in their families. Third, she suggests that because many of the older women have themselves been 'experts' in caring work, for example looking after their own families in their own homes, finding themselves in situations in which they are dependent on other women is extremely difficult. This is a form of assault on their identity, in which they are effectively forced to surrender, in whole or in part, their ownership of care work to other women. Finally, she contends that many of the nurses actually found caring for older women threatening to who they are as women themselves. On the one hand, both groups see themselves as 'expert carers', and this can set up tensions. On the other hand, and of fundamental importance to our concerns here, she argues that the female nurses are daily confronted with images of what they themselves might become in the future: frail older women. In this situation, they operate strategies which enable them to distance themselves to a degree from their female patients – and, by extension, from growing older – as a means of maintaining their own integrity and sense of self.

In the second study, our colleague Gillian Granville (1992) used Evers's work as a basis for her Masters dissertation, which examined how female health visitors saw their role with older women. In depth tape-recorded interviews with fifteen health visitors revealed that most of them were reactive rather than proactive in their work with older women. Moreover, Granville (1992) also found that most of them tended passively to accept women's role as informal carers in the private domain and saw health visiting as simply a professional extension of this identity. As in the work by Evers (1981), being confronted with a possible future image of themselves was unnerving, and none of them saw ageing in a positive way. In fact, six interviewees did not even want to think about ageing, viewing it with fear and apprehension. The other nine talked about how they planned to be as healthy as they could in their own old age and were making financial plans and adopting healthier lifestyles as their way of dealing with the future. But, what was particularly disturbing was that, although many of them were knowledgeable about the importance of adopting healthy lifestyles, this was only directed at improving their own health rather than towards helping the older women with whom they worked.

It is instructive to note that these two empirical studies also contain echoes of much of the feminist research on informal caring that was carried out in the latter half of the 1980s. For example, the in-depth study of nineteen carers in Canterbury by Clare Ungerson (1987) examined the ways in which both men and women try to make sense of the caring that they do. Her sample contained six women who were caring for their own mothers and a further three who were caring for their mothers-in-law. Like Evers (1981), Ungerson's (1987) work highlights the stresses around role reversal experienced by many of the women who cared for their mothers or mothers-in-law. They talk about how they can only care for their mothers and mothers-in-law if they cut themselves off from feelings (i.e. from caring *about* someone) and get on with the tasks involved (i.e. simply concentrated on caring *for* their relative). They also talk about how they cope by ignoring their feelings or by burying them; if they do not do this, the strength of their emotions prevents them from carrying out essential personal tasks. Ungerson also draws attention to the conflicts and rivalry between these different generations of women concerning the home and women's traditional domestic domain.

These themes also feature in a larger study carried out by Jane Lewis and Barbara Meredith (1988). They conducted intensive interviews with forty-one daughters who had been co-resident carers of their mothers but who, at the time that they were interviewed, had ceased to care because their mother had either died or gone into institutional care. These daughters too had difficulties in dealing with what they saw as a process of role reversal (a number had very dominant and possessive mothers). By way of response, many of them adopted a variety of techniques to distance themselves from their mothers. Some would treat her as a different person: 'that little old lady, not mum'; some would infantilise her, treating her as another child or baby; some regarded mother as a 'case' to be dealt with; some would ensure a certain amount of 'geographical distance' within the home in terms of territory or closing the bedroom door; and some would actively plan for the future when 'mum' would no longer be there.

Crucially, too, Lewis and Meredith (1988) observed that some carers experienced considerable difficulties in coming to terms with their own ageing and were fearful of it. They were faced, as in Evers's study, with an image of their mother's deteriorating health. Indeed, they had to live with it on a day-to-day basis, and for those whose mothers were suffering from Alzheimer's disease this proved particularly difficult. Again though, individual responses to this situation would vary. Some daughters recognised that their own fears led to them perhaps being overprotective of their mothers to the detriment of their own well-being. Others found that this heightened their awareness of the ways in which older people were treated by society and resolved to confront and challenge, as far as possible, the stereotypes of themselves as they age. Lewis and Meredith (1988: 71) quite rightly caution us that we need to understand fully the 'complicated dynamic' that characterises mother–daughter relationships if we are to ensure that appropriate support is offered which is acceptable to both the carer and the cared-for person. We would suggest that such a caution is no less valid to our current considerations in this chapter.

It appears then that, while we can cull points of interest from the existing literature, there is a sense that much is still unknowable and unknown about women's experiences of ageing. There are however some key areas which have been identified, including the connections to be made between ageing and identity (and the possible centrality of work identity for many professional women); the fear and apprehension with which ageing and older women still seem to be viewed, even by women who are themselves ageing; and the tensions and complexities that the interplay of these individual and societal themes sets up for women who are themselves the professional carers of other older women. Thus, to illustrate some of these issues, we turn now to findings from our own research and practice.

Reflections on growing older

The material that we draw on comes first from an exploratory study in which participants at a major conference on nursing and older people were requested to complete a brief questionnaire titled 'Reflections on ageing'. The intention was to consider what might be problematic or difficult about ageing for a particular group of professional women, alongside the positive and creative potential that ageing and old age may present us with. Second, the emergent themes from this study are then further illustrated using vignettes drawn from counselling practice. Our intention here is not to examine the benefits or otherwise of counselling *per se*, but simply to use these examples as ways of amplifying some of the issues about ageing with which mid-life women juggle daily. Great care has been taken to preserve the anonymity of these women and all have given permission to use their material.

Forty-one women delegates to the conference returned completed questionnaires, of whom twenty-seven (66%) were aged in their forties or fifties. These twenty-seven women all worked directly with older people in hospitals (in continuing care, rehabilitation, general medicine, dementia units), in the independent sector (in nursing or dual registered homes) or in the community. Not surprisingly, many of them had worked with older people for a considerable length of time: on average, for 11 years, although some had spent their entire careers in this field. The vast majority (twenty-three or 85%) were registered general nurses or state registered nurses. Moreover, nearly one-third of them (eight or 30%) also had a first degree, while three (11%) had a specialist higher degree (MA or MSc) in gerontology and two (7%) women had a university diploma in nursing. In addition, seven (26%) women possessed teaching qualifications (certificate in education, registered nurse tutor), three (11%) were registered mental health nurses, two (7%) had management qualifications (MBA, CMS) and another two (7%) had undertaken English National Board courses of various kinds. Between them, they also possessed a whole gamut of certificates and diplomas, including some for health education, counselling, herbalism, massage and orthopaedic nursing.

These twenty-seven women all completed sentence stems concerning what they most feared about ageing and about being an old woman. Not one woman responded by saying there was nothing she feared. Rather, four very clear themes emerged, which were concerned with:

- ill health;
- dependency;
- loneliness;
- identity, dignity and appearance.

These four themes are now each discussed in turn below.

Ill health

Many of the respondents to the questionnaire completed the sentence stems with reference to the biological and health changes that they feared ageing would bring. They said, 'the things I most fear about ageing are':

- ill health preventing me doing things;
- being disabled mentally, physically or both;
- not being in control of my mind.

None of the women actually mentioned death but, as we see below in the vignette about Anne, the actual experience of ill health in mid- or later life (as opposed to just its future possibility) often has close links with thoughts about one's own ageing and mortality.

Anne, a lecturer in her mid-fifties, had once again been diagnosed as having cancer. Ten years previously, she had had a mastectomy and had undergone a course of chemotherapy. Now, still in mid-life, she was faced with what she termed 'a repeat performance'. Although she knew what to expect, her fears around facing the pain and the inevitable physical disfigurement were exacerbated by the fact that this time she would have to face it alone. Her husband, who had supported her on the previous occasion, had since died and there was no one else. During the unfolding of her story, she admitted that she was less afraid of dying than she was of living and ageing with disfigurement and illness. She had hoped that she might meet someone with whom to share the rest of her life, but now, given her impending physical condition, she felt the prospect of that happening was virtually impossible. Over the months after her operation, Anne spent a good deal of her time engaging in what she described as 'meaning of life' activities: she read extensively; engaged in meditation, sometimes alone and at other times with a group of like-minded people; and she continued writing her personal journal. She decided to take time out and focus her attention on what she described as the inner healing process. Anne's despair about the prospect of what she anticipated was in store propelled her into intensifying her search for the meaning of life and, in the process, she took charge of her life and herself in order to do so.

Dependency

Closely linked with fears about ill health and about one's own mortality are concerns about how long we might be able to remain independent. In this context, respondents noted that 'the things I most fear about ageing are':

- losing my independence;
- being dependent on others for personal care;
- becoming a burden to my family and society.

Margaret's vignette clearly illustrates the salience of these fears for some professional women, as well as demonstrating the close interrelationship between the themes of dependency and ill health.

Margaret had taken early retirement from the teaching profession approximately 6 years before she sought counselling. She had become increasingly debilitated by her arthritic condition and was in a state of great distress, despair and anger. Her greatest fears were that she would become, as her mother had before her, confined to a wheelchair, isolated and totally dependent upon others. Margaret had cared for her mother for a while, but eventually decided, because of her own professional commitments, that she should go into a nursing home to be cared for. Margaret vividly remembered the environment in which her mother spent her final days and dreaded such a prospect for herself. Here then was a woman now battling with the conflict of dependence versus independence as she herself aged.

She firmly believed that having to take early retirement had had an adverse effect upon her socially, psychologically and physically. Had she taken ample time planning for her retirement, she believes she would have managed it much more productively. Despite her arthritis having taken its toll in that her body was visibly distorted and her mobility adversely affected, she described her physical self as 'an inconvenient challenge'. Of much greater importance to her was the fact that she experienced herself as useful and independent. She wanted to prolong her active life in her own community, was realistic about the positive effects of occasional outside care and gradually began to make moves towards part-time voluntary work. She was determined to work with what was happening rather than let it dictate to her, although she recognised some of the ambivalences, and even denial of ageing, that still remained.

Loneliness

We might hypothesise that reflections about dependency and ill-health embody an awareness that these are more likely to be concomitants of ageing for women, while at the same time underscoring the dominant, problem-orientated and negative images we have of old age. To these, we can add our third theme: feelings of loneliness. A number of respondents to the questionnaire replied that 'the things I most fear about ageing are':

- loneliness;
- loneliness because I have no siblings or children;
- the long lonely minutes when all my past mistakes will have time to haunt me.

Greta, a community nurse, was aged 60 and had been widowed for approximately 6 months when she was referred for counselling. She was in a state of great despair and was unable to make any sense of her life without her husband. They had done almost everything together before his death and neither of them had socialised with people living nearby. The few friends with whom they had kept in contact were people they had known since their teenage years, before they were married. These 'old' friends lived a long way away and Greta had no heart to contact them. She had stopped looking after herself properly, was not eating well, had no motivation to cook or go shopping and had no interest in how she looked. She felt totally alone and had, in a very real sense, lost her identity and her dignity. In her very isolated world, she appeared dull, almost lifeless. Her skin had a grey appearance, her hair was dishevelled and her clothes dowdy. She said she had no mission in life anymore. Over the months, her general appearance became 'lighter': she no longer slouched, she walked taller and with a sense of purpose and she wore clothes which enhanced her appearance. Much of

Greta's despair and loneliness was clearly linked with having no one with whom to share her thoughts about her deceased partner, about life before the death, the dying process and her present feelings about ageing and the losses that she was experiencing.

Identity, dignity and appearance

Our fourth and final theme brings together the essence of the fears that many mid-life women have about ageing. Ageing is accompanied, in the minds of many respondents to the questionnaire, by concerns about changes to one's identity and self-image and, importantly, to one's physical appearance. They said, 'the things I most fear about ageing are':

- having wrinkles and looking ugly;
- losing my hair, being useless and losing my sense of self;
- being disregarded, becoming invisible, being seen as an asexual being;
- being stereotyped, abused and unrespected;
- younger people seeing me as old and unable.

Helen, a woman in her early fifties, had been a teacher until her children left home and she decided to retire from the teaching profession to undertake a full-time higher degree course at the local university. Half-way through the course, her husband, a successful businessman, became incapacitated as a result of a serious accident and Helen felt obliged to discontinue her studies in order to look after him. Helen was very concerned that her husband's condition in some way mirrored what happens to us all when we get too old to look after ourselves. She would pass observations such as: 'Well, I could be like that some day myself, when I'm old and grey.' She also worried about what the future held for her and wondered if she was destined for ever for what she described as the lifeless life she was now living. At other times, she would announce that she was surely not too old to want more from life than this.

After some time and much agonising, Helen arrived at a compromise. She decided to employ a professional carer for her husband for part of the week. She enrolled on a new part-time course of study and made an effort to join in some of the social events associated with the course.

These brief vignettes graphically portray some of the feelings about ageing and becoming an older woman that were highlighted in the opening pages of this chapter and in the empirical work of both Evers (1981) and Granville (1992). These women all exhibit, in varying ways and in differing combinations, the range of fears associated with ageing, such as ill health, dependency, loneliness and changes to one's identity, dignity and appearance.

What these women share is their gender and their status as professional women. Many also have considerable experience of work with older people. Yet, ageing is viewed with trepidation: it is perceived as bringing with it negative changes to one's identity and self-image; to one's physical appearance; and to one's ability to exercise control and choice over oneself and one's surroundings. Even in the unique stories that each woman brings to counselling, they all spend a great deal of time discussing the ageing process and how this affects their personal and professional lives. Their comments illustrate the complex interplay and impact of both age and gender: what has eloquently been termed the 'double standard of ageing' by Susan Sontag (1978), whereby women are not permitted to age in ways that men are. Perhaps the fears of many mid-life women are best summed up in the words of one 48-year-old nurse who wrote on her questionnaire that: 'The things I most fear about ageing are…losing my mind, losing my looks, and losing my front door key.'

Looking forward

Although women who seek counselling have, understandably, come at a particularly problematic or crucial juncture in their lives, behind their stories are hints that ageing itself, and reflecting on the process and changes it brings, may not be wholly negative. Anne talked at length about the opportunity her illness gave her to take stock of her life, to reappraise her lifestyle and get more in touch with her spiritual self. Margaret's goal was to be able to plan for the future and to continue to find pleasure in the voluntary work that she is now able to do. Greta is coming through her despair and depression and meeting the future with a renewed understanding of who she is. Helen, too, has come to a recognition that she needs people and is making an effort to do things that she has previously struggled to do, such as socialising.

These positive reflections were also echoed in the responses to the questionnaire from the twenty-seven nurses. They completed sentence stems about what they most looked forward to about ageing and three major, but closely interrelated, themes emerged. They looked forward to ageing for 'family' reasons; for the 'time and freedom' it would bring; and for the opportunity it afforded to 'be oneself'. Some of the comments they made about each of these areas were as follows.

Family and children
- to be able to see my children and several generations to come;
- enjoying my family and appreciating their achievements;

- spending time with my grandchildren; and being a grandmother.

Time, freedom and activity
- doing the things I do not have time for now;
- having time to participate more in life within my community;
- having less responsibility and more freedom;
- being able to indulge in all those activities which work and family never allowed time for; doing all the things I could not do when younger – starting new ventures; gaining experiences, maturity, confidence and skills.

Being oneself
- having more time to be myself;
- losing the worries of middle age and having time to be me;
- I can be as outrageous as I like, wear what I want, get fat if I want;
- not caring about what other people think.

These comments illustrate some of the strengths and opportunities that age may bring. Alongside their trepidation, these women recognise the possibilities for continued self-development and creativity beyond the pressures of work and domestic responsibilities. They also demonstrate what we know from research about the importance of family ties, social support and social networks to women as they age. Women's instrumental and affective ties are viewed as strengths to be built upon (Sheila Peace, 1986; Alice Rossi, 1986; Dorothy Jerrome, 1993). In the words of one respondent:

> The things I most look forward to about ageing are…not having to worry about working and looking after others' needs, but enjoying being a grandmother, being able to continue to write poetry, and to share ideas, reflections and my life experiences with family and friends.

Our ageing selves

By way of conclusion to this chapter, we offer here some final comments about the material that we have presented and discussed above. As women who are ageing, mid-life professionals such as ourselves need to take stock of, and discuss, these issues. At the end of their first book, *Growing Old Disgracefully*, members of the Hen Co-Op (1993) ask the question: 'Do you want to grow old disgracefully with other like-minded women?' The authors, together with the publishers of the book, have established a loose-knit national network of women interested in exploring this whole area. Those of us who work in and alongside the caring professions might usefully be encouraged to create similar networks and opportunities in order to examine what it means to be part and parcel of the ageing enterprise. The generation of our own Keele Women's Gerontology Group was originally designed to do just this. Twice a year, the group would plan a whole day's workshop to continue to explore and debate aspects of growing older, as it affected both our professional and personal lives. Although this was an absorbing and stimulating way to spend a Saturday, it was interesting that such a group felt the need to travel from all over the country to meet together to discuss and debate these issues. While participation in the gerontology course was a common and binding thread, it is notable that this kind of support and openness appeared, at the time, to be missing within individuals' own work environments or personal networks.

This in turn leads us to conclude that not only do we need to look more closely at ageing as it affects our lives as mid-life professional women, but that we also need to work with and for older women in our professional capacities and to engage in discussion and debate with them. Instead of perpetuating an 'us' and 'them' mentality, we must consciously begin to make links between 'us', the 'ageing women', and 'them', the 'aged women'. This logically begins, as in this chapter, with our own reflections about ageing, but needs then to extend to a critical analysis of current practices and attitudes, which also incorporate the views and opinions of older women themselves. Whether we like it or not, mid-life and older women reflect inescapable mirror images of each other. However, the mirror image is something we need to work with, not ignore. Although, as we have shown, comparatively little empirical work yet addresses how mid-life women feel about and deal with their own ageing, we believe it is an area worthy of further exploration and research for at least three reasons: first, it would begin to make visible some of the complexity, tensions and potential for women in this period of their mature adulthood and would add their voice to the literature; second, it would help bridge the gap which undoubtedly exists between the, as yet, mostly gender-neutral theoretical discourses about mid-life and ageing (see, for example, Biggs, 1999a) and how this is played out in reality for women; third, it would offer some further insights into the ways in which mid-life professional women's own understandings of ageing may or may not have an impact on their interactions with the older women for whom they care.

It is appropriate therefore to conclude this chapter with the unequivocal words of the radical lesbian feminist Baba Copper (1988: 86–7), who tells us that:

> …there are ways that all women can begin to prepare the way for the empowerment of themselves in the future, when they are old… The

first step is for women to recognize that they have been programmed to hate old women and to deny them power. This brainwashing is so subtle that its eradication will take an effort equal to that which we have made and still must make upon sexism. Further, this brainwashing extends through our lives, making us fear the processes of our own bodies within time. These are attitudes and expectations which we can change if we decide to. Empowerment of women will come when we identify with women older than we are and not before.

5   Menopause

A time of private change to a mature identity

Gillian Granville

Introduction

Menopause has been the subject of an intense public debate throughout the 1980s and 1990s and has had an impact on the cohort of women known as the 'baby boomers', who are currently in mid-life. Two polarised discourses concerning the menopause experience have dominated debates: one is located in a biomedical model and the other within a radical feminist framework. The medical response has been to construct menopause as a deficiency disease, requiring treatment in order to prevent illnesses in old age such as osteoporosis and Alzheimer's disease. It is clearly defined in biomedical language with signs and symptoms, stages through the process and medical interventions, the most significant of which is hormone replacement therapy (HRT). The opposing radical feminist response has been to critique the biomedical model, suggesting that it is part of a conspiracy by men and male-dominated institutions to control women's ageing at mid-life. It rejects the need for treatment, promoting the view that women should see menopause as a natural event in the life-course which can liberate them from the oppressive nature of men (Germaine Greer, 1991; Sandra Coney, 1995).

However, contemporary feminists are now seeking new ways to interpret the experience of menopause, using psychodynamic and post-modernist/post-structuralist frameworks. It is in this context that the present chapter focuses on results from an empirical study of twenty 'baby boomer' women who are now approaching mid-life. In the study, I sought to understand the meanings that mid-life women place on the experience of menopause. As a feminist myself, and a member of the same cohort, I was acutely aware of the need to adopt a reflexive approach and to understand critically how my individual experience may impinge on the research process. The work is thus set within a contemporary feminist framework, influenced both by gerontological theories and by the psychodynamic tradition. The chapter begins with a more detailed exposition of the current literature on menopause before going on to explain the way that I hoped to ensure the voices of women were heard through the application of feminist methodology. The chapter then concentrates on some of the findings, demonstrating how women view menopause as a transition to a mature identity and how, in the process of change, they became aware of the hostile social world that older women inhabit.

Current discourses on menopause

A *deficiency disease*

It was in the late 1960s that menopause began to be defined as a deficiency disease as a result, in part, of the influence of the Canadian gynaecologist Robert Wilson. His book *Feminine Forever* (Wilson, 1966) has this description on the cover: 'a fully-documented discussion of one of medicine's most revolutionary breakthroughs – the discovery that menopause is a hormone deficient disease, curable and preventable'. He also suggested that the unpalatable truth that needed to be faced was that all post-menopausal women are castrates. Constructed within a biomedical framework, the menopause has signs and symptoms of illness which can be treated. The medical literature gives only three agreed symptoms: altered menstrual flow, genital atrophy (thinning of the skin and dryness) and vasomotor symptoms (hot flushes and night sweats) (Wilson, 1995). These symptoms are commonly discussed in the medical and academic literature, in health information leaflets and in the media, along with other possible, but not universally agreed, symptoms such as depression, insomnia, headaches, itchy skin, joint pains and loss of libido. Jean Ginsburg (1992) produced a table that was ranked in order of prevalence of symptoms, from 70% for hot flushes to 12% for swollen ankles, although she does not specify how this information was collected and from which women. However, she does state:

> Whilst it is difficult to link every single symptom specifically to the menopause, a surprising number are reasonably attributable to oestrogen deficiency. Menopausal hot flushes wake the woman from sleep, and oestrogen deprivation has been shown to be associated with a characteristic change in the electroencephalogram, both of which are restored to normal when menopausal women are treated with oestrogens.
>
> (Ginsburg, 1992: 104)

Once menopause became defined as a disease, women were regarded as sick and in need of treatment. The body was deficient in oestrogen and by giving women hormone replacement therapy they would be restored to their previous premenopausal state. Its use is also promoted for short-term relief of menopausal symptoms and for the prevention of illnesses in old age, such as osteoporosis, heart disease and Alzheimer's disease. However, there are conflicting reports about the uptake of HRT among women. Previous statistics (cited in Coney, 1995: 172) put the figure at 30% of American women using it compared with 10% of British and Australian women. In Britain, sales for HRT totalled £10 million by 1989, doubling sales figures in 2 years, and it was estimated that by the year 2000 one-quarter of British women would be using it. Madge Vickers (1997) reported that world-wide one in five women aged between 50 and 64 take hormone replacements, but this did not indicate the number of women who stop taking it without telling their doctor.

Although it may be difficult to obtain accurate figures, it is clear that, at the turn of the century, there has not been the comprehensive take up that was anticipated, in spite of continual attempts by the pharmaceutical companies to promote and develop oestrogen replacements. Frances Griffiths's (1995a) survey of 1,697 British women aged between 20 and 69 years found that the use and promotion of hormone replacement therapy for prevention appears to be relatively unimportant for women when taken in the context of the total health and welfare of the community. The survey also indicated that 'the widespread fear of cancer may affect women's attitudes to hormone replacement therapy, even when the risk of breast cancer proves to be extremely small' (Griffiths, 1995b: 58).

The links between breast cancer and the use of HRT remain one of the most contentious issues in medical literature and generate considerable research (see, for example, Bergkvist *et al.*, 1989; Colditz *et al.*, 1993). It has also stimulated the need for comprehensive longitudinal studies to examine the preventive claims of the treatment. The WISDOM international project, for example, was established in 1997 to chart the health of some 34,000 women taking HRT or an inactive placebo (dummy) tablet for 10 years and who are to be followed up for a further 10 years (Vickers, 1997). This is an example of a randomised controlled trial which, in scientific research terms, is considered to be the conclusive way that definitive answers are found (Susan Love, 1997) and is typical of the biomedical approach's favoured method of research. Other large-scale studies include the 'Million Women Study', a UK national survey being carried out at the Radcliffe Infirmary, Oxford, which is collecting information by anonymous, self-completion questionnaire of women attending for breast screening. Also, in 1991, the Women's Health Initiative, Bethesda, USA, began a 10-year controlled study of 140,000 middle-aged and older women to examine the effects of dietary and hormone therapy and treatment on menopause and specific disease processes (see Colette Browne, 1998: 200).

A natural event

The radical feminist challenge to the biomedical construction of menopause spans two decades and has largely been concentrated in Australian and North American literature (see Rosetta Reitz, 1987; Jean Shapiro, 1989; Greer, 1991). Its principal argument is to reject totally menopause as a hormone-deficient disease which requires treatment and, instead, to contextualise it as a natural experience in the life-course of women. Germaine Greer (1991), whose work has been particularly influential, defines the menopause as a natural event which offers women a time of spiritual reawakening, rebirth, rehabilitation and a release from the sexual attention of men. She feels sorry for women who take hormone replacement therapy and are denied this opportunity to have serenity and peace, further suggesting that: 'The climacteric marks the end of apologising. The chrysalis of conditioning has once and for all to break and the female woman finally emerges' (Greer, 1991: 440).

Greer has not been without her feminist critics in the way that she believes that menopause is natural and that all women should welcome it as they grow older. Some feel that the emphasis on 'natural' minimises women's experiences of mid-life (see Komesaroff *et al.*, 1997; Lyn Richards *et al.*, 1997). Lyn Richards regards a denial of the need to be young and attractive in a youth-orientated society as grave simplification and, as a card-carrying feminist, 'I'm having trouble with it' (Richards *et al.*, 1997: 102). Kwok Wei Leng (1997) talks of the only two options that seem to be available for mid-life women: to accept hormone replacement therapy and be dubbed a victim of patriarchy or to resist it and believe in the body and restore power to the crone.

A patriarchal conspiracy

Other feminist critiques of the biomedical interpretation of menopause challenged the consumerist approach, in which products and services are targeted at mid-life women and play on a belief that women fear growing old. Nancy Worcester and Marian Whatley (1992), for example, questioned the sudden interest in older women's health issues, such as osteoporosis and heart disease, after decades of ignoring them. They believe that this raised awareness is directly related to the medical establishment and the drug industry's 'discovery' that healthy, menopausal and post-menopausal women present a huge market for their products. Sandra Coney (1995) describes a conspiracy between the medical profession and pharmaceutical companies, which sets out to exploit women at mid-life. Her arguments track the discovery of hormone replacement therapy in the 1970s, when it was recommended for women with menopausal symptoms for a short time span, to what she interprets as the sinister changes that took place in the late 1980s, when it was marketed for lifetime use as a prevention of disease in old age. She argues that the drug companies have made profits out of experimenting with women's lives and describes how they seek to influence doctors to prescribe their products.

Women's experiences across cultures

The feminist response to the disease model of menopause has been argued, until recently, from within a radical feminist framework, but with very little in the way of empirical studies to support it. Previously, women's experiences were to be found in a small body of social anthropological and ethnographic studies which construct menopause as a universal event in the lives of women with different cultural and historical expressions. One of the dominant themes in the sociocultural model is that positive individual and societal attitudes towards ageing and old women lead to a diminishing or absence of menopausal symptoms (see, for example, Dona Davies, 1989; Flint and Samil, 1990; Moore and Kombe, 1991; Lock, 1993; Martin *et al.*, 1993; Chirawatkul and Manderson, 1994; Gabriella Berger, 1999). Such cross-cultural research, Marsha Carolan (1994) suggests, illustrates the connections between cultural values and assumptions and prevailing health experiences. It contests the view of menopause as a hormone-deficient disease by contrasting Western women's experiences with those of women from other cultures. However, Carolan (1994: 200) warns that: 'it may be impossible to separate the "purely" physiological from the cultural as they are necessarily intertwined'. This theme has been developed in Gabriella Berger's (1999) work, in which she attempts to conceptualise the impact of cultural beliefs by arguing that they come from three elements: women's roles, women's bodies and the ageing process. The relationship of these three form the physical, psychological and social experiences of menopause. She found no evidence to support a symptoms checklist and even the hot flush had no consistency when examined cross-culturally: 'Menopause, this transient and mystical phase, advances often in secret without a woman's knowledge, leaving no visible traces' (Berger, 1999:182).

The sociocultural critique of the biomedical model has enabled menopause to be situated within experiences other than those of a predominantly white American, middle-class context. It has also assisted the development of an increasing body of theoretical and empirical work which is concerned with women's experiences of menopause and its links to ageing and mid-life. Some of the theoretical understanding of this is to be found in post-modern discourses, in which feminists are contributing to the growing intellectual uncertainty about the appropriate grounding and methods for explaining and interpreting women's experiences (Ruth Ray,

1996). Contemporary feminist research is exploring new ways that menopause can be understood in an effort to establish new paradigms grounded in women's experiences of the social world that they inhabit (Geri Dickson, 1993; Sandra Cross and Joseph Lovett, 1994).

New paradigms

The post-modern literature criticises feminist arguments for being on the same side as the biomedical ones (see Patricia Kaufert, 1982; Davis, 1989; Emily Martin, 1993; Komesaroff *et al.*, 1997). Both positions are filled, post-modernists argue, with assumptions about the world and the feminists' 'normal body' and the patriarchs' 'medicalised body' are equally constructed forms of the same discourse. Kwok Wei Leng (1997: 264) believes that:

> It seems that the classical feminist writings on menopause have thus far contained fundamental similarities to the biomedical writings on menopause. Both models operate as closed thought-systems...the feminist model shares with the biomedical model the same philosophical assumptions about truth. It seems that the great divide between the two positions turns out to be no divide at all, but rather two sides of the same coin.

Post-modernists are seeking to understand the meaning of menopause in terms of a physiological transition that all women will experience, but with a great deal of individual variation. Emily Martin (1993) suggests that through menstruation, menopause and childbirth a woman's body in medical texts is organised as a hierarchical system. Inherent in this concept is the mind controlling the body. She claims that, by separating the body and mind, it is possible to move away from the negative aspects of biological determinism.

Carmel Seibold (1997), in her study of twenty, single mid-life women, found the opposite to this view in that women were striving for a sense of wholeness rather than a separation of mind and body. She found the relationship that women had with their bodies before mid-life affected their response to their ageing and menopausal body. She concluded:

> I contend that the body is the centre of this [wholeness] for women throughout their lives; whether it is attempting to ignore it as a celibate woman, controlling fertility as partnered women, or controlling it and making it work as a mid-life and menopausal woman. The strongest message to emerge from the women in this study was a sense of striving in mid-life for wholeness and integration: the body becoming my body.
> (Seibold, 1997: 76)

Jacquelyn Zita (1993) also suggests that the body is an object which acquires social meaning and social location through cultural practices, and that the construction of the menopausal body using imagery signifying shame and disempowerment makes it easier to deny the potential power of the old woman. These links to self-identity and the physical experience of the menopausal body are stimulating research which seeks to understand the rules and meanings that frame women's lives and experiences. One such approach attempts to examine critically menopause as a transition, or marker, that enables women to consider their position in the life-course.

A marker of growth or decline

Menopause is frequently referred to in the popular media and the academic literature as a transition (see, for example, Reitz, 1987; Coope, 1996; Fiona Mackie, 1997), carrying with it the implication of changing from one state, or set of circumstances, to another. Hence, the popular use of the term 'the change'. Transition also suggests that there is a recognisable event and one which irrevocably changes a woman's life (Richards *et al.*, 1997); in the biomedical literature, menopause distinguishes between the reproductive and non-reproductive parts of a woman's life. More recently, Margaret Gullette (1997) has argued that the menopause has been socially constructed as a 'magic marker' of decline, whereas Gail Sheehy (1994, 1997) terms menopause a 'silent passage', from which women re-emerge in their fifties with a high level of well-being and inner harmony. However, with the exception of the work of Australian researchers Lyn Richards, Carmel Seibold and Nicole Davis (1997), there is currently little empirical evidence, particularly from the UK, which is able to validate these contentions. Consequently, my own study, reported here, is one attempt to understand women's experiences of the menopause and ageing through their own narratives.

Seeking to understand women's experiences

The study developed out of my own interest as a feminist, reaching mid-life and being acutely conscious in the early 1990s of the public debate surrounding menopause and hormone replacement therapy. The media appeared to focus attention on white, middle-class married women with children who had grown up and left home. However, I knew from my own experience and observations that the lives of women are more diverse than these narrow stereotypes allowed, and I was curious to know whether women's experience of menopause was different and individual to them or whether there was a collective meaning which could be assigned to it.

I chose to use a feminist methodological approach because I wished to ground the research process in a feminist theoretical framework (Shulamit Reinharz, 1992). I wanted to use feminist theory to design, conduct and analyse the process and I wanted the findings to contribute and feed back into feminist and gerontological thinking. First then, the research is guided by feminist theory and, in particular, by an examination of the interaction of gender and power. Second, the experiences of women are central to the research process, inform the outcomes and point the way forward for new research agendas. Third, the women who tell their stories are empowered by the process to varying degrees. Finally, I, as the researcher, am located in the process in a number of ways: I am in the same age group as the participating women and we shared personal experiences during the interview. I kept a reflexive diary, so I was conscious of how I may be influencing the research through my own reflexive gaze (Steier, 1991).

The study involved semistructured interviews with twenty women, who were all aged between 45 and 50 and who were living in the West Midlands. Different approaches were taken to access the women. Certain women were known to me, whereas other 'hard to reach' groups, for example lesbian women, were accessed through an intermediary. They were not extraordinary women in society's terms, but they had all led lives that showed the challenges and oppressive practices that women face daily. Moreover, the richness of diversity is reflected in a number of ways. My sample included women with a range of educational opportunities and paid work experiences, such as a scientist, a worker in the arts, a cup handler in a pottery factory and women doing piece-work in a factory distribution plant. Some participants worked as professional women in education, health and social services, whereas another was in the family business. In socioeconomic terms, some women described themselves as from a privileged background, while others came from more deprived ones. One woman was an identical twin; some were black women from Africa and the Caribbean who spent their formative years in racist societies. Another woman has lived most of her life with the aid of a wheelchair, and another has been profoundly deaf since the age of 2 years. Two women referred to themselves as gay in their sexual orientation and were happy to share the effect that this has had on their lives. The place of child-bearing and child-rearing also challenged the stereotypes of women, with some women choosing to stay childless, another having a child in her forties, some in paid work alongside their role as mothers and others choosing to bring up a child alone. Many were also caring for or supporting older relatives in a variety of ways.

At the beginning of the study, I had been strongly influenced by the radical feminist analysis of the biomedical model of menopause and by my own experiences of working with, and being part of, the 'baby boomer' cohort. I sought confirmation that there was a patriarchal conspiracy against older women which put them in competition with each other. However, as my analysis progressed and I listened closely to the women's words, I became aware of a different voice emerging from their accounts. At this stage, I decided to put the literature to one side and adopt a grounded approach to the data (Layder, 1993) which enabled me to identify emerging themes from the women's narratives. Here, I concentrate in particular on themes relating to temporality, to the changing private self and to the impact of the public gaze.

Menopause as a time of change

One of the emerging themes from the data was the concept of temporality in which the women understood menopause as a time in the life-course which they moved through and which led to a changed sense of themselves. The work of Glaser and Strauss (1971) on status passage was a useful framework in which to interpret the women's words, and showed how women entered, paused, moved forward and then emerged from this mid-life transition.

Entering the change

Alterations in the cyclical rhythm of their bodies and the final cessation of menstruation was only one of the markers that the women used to recognise they had entered a transition. In my study, four of the women had ceased menstruating in their early forties, either naturally or through hysterectomy, but still considered themselves to be menopausal at around the age of 50. This also appears to relate to the importance in the life-course of 'on-time' or 'off-time' age experiences (see, for example, Neugarten, 1968; Sara Arber and Jay Ginn, 1995). Joy did not feel that she was experiencing a biological menopause because she was still having periods but, when I asked her to describe what she meant by menopause, she replied: 'Women in their 50s. I should say ageing women, but it is just women in their 50s, mid-50s'. I discussed this reply with Joy when I revisited her with her transcript and she said that she had thought a great deal about the response since the initial interview, and, yes, that was indeed what it meant to her, 'ageing women'. Joan also made a link between age and menopause when we were talking about reaching 50 (Joan was 49 and was still having regular periods). She thought reaching 50 was quite a 'landmark', and then went on to say:

> Yes, I think so because, well I think it is, because with women, with perhaps the menopause and going through that, I think it is because it is a very obvious change, not obvious to the outside world, but obvious to yourself. It is telling you that you are going into an older age isn't it?

The women were also aware that, in British society, there is no public ritual to mark formally the beginning or end of menstruation and its association with fertility, and therefore no easily recognisable rite of passage into another part of life. Joyce, who came to England from Africa in the 1960s, spoke about the rituals associated with menstruation in her culture when there were traditional gatherings as a celebration of your 'womanhood'. However, there was no such occasion for menopause:

> You see, we celebrate the fertility years at home but there is no ritual about menopause. Why not? There should be a ritual about not having to use contraceptives, not having to have so many babies.
>
> (Joyce)

In spite of this lack of public acknowledgement, many of the women recognised themselves as privately entering a changing period of their lives. They demonstrated, at times, a state described by Glaser and Strauss (1971: 37) as 'closed awareness', when there is a hesitation or level of uncertainty about whether a transition has been entered and a degree of 'wait and see' is required. Claire was telling me about the reactions of her husband when she began the menopause:

> I don't think he was very understanding at the beginning until he talked to his work friend, and his wife was similar. Because...sort of...twelve months ago, I went through a phase [pause] where I had got [sigh] really, really depressed and low, and I think that was another start of it [menopause].

Claire is identifying a certain time, looking back, when she entered a transition by her use of words such as 'beginning' and 'start'. Similarly, it was only when Milly looked back that she realised she had entered the menopause because she had not associated the hot sensations that she was experiencing with hot flushes: 'I didn't realise at first when my hot flushes were starting. I suppose it would be about 18 months ago when I realised because they were happening very often.'

Some women anticipated entering a transition, even before they had reached it. Julia talked of a naturally occurring process and demonstrated the inevitability of it by saying:

> Well I don't think it is a disease, it is a natural process, and it is not an illness, it is a natural process. It is something that, perhaps it is not worth worrying about. If I say it is not worth worrying about, that indicates that you can't take anything to help it or stop ageing. But,

there is no point in getting yourself worked up, like there is no point getting yourself worked up about dying because it is going to happen at the end. So I can't, I can't get worked up about the menopause because it is going to happen, so you just have to accept it and get on with it.

Permission to pause

The menopause transition was interpreted from many of the women's narratives as a time in the life-course when they could pause to reflect on themselves, before moving forward into a new phase of their lives. Jasmine had recently had a career which she had given up for health reasons, as well as making other adjustments to her personal life. She considered that she was experiencing menopausal symptoms, but also demonstrated the way she was re-evaluating her life at this time in the life-course:

I try not to look ahead too much and at one point I was getting quite negative over the arthritis, but I see it as a very exciting time actually, because I think I am actually, I have diversified away from [one career to another], and I think I am now where I should be. It is something I have come to. I just believe that your life is set out in front of you anyway, and I can see how my life, I can see the stepping stones in my life, that have taken me, which have brought me, to where I am now.

This was a strong and consistent theme in the narratives: that now was the opportunity to stand back, take stock and decide on how they wished to lead the rest of their lives. The individual circumstances were all different, from the women who had suffered from society's prejudices of race, disability and sexual orientation to those women suffering less overt oppression in difficult relationships and financial hardship. They were considering what had gone before, reflecting on how they had reached this point in the life-course and how they could manage future roles which were right for them. Joan planned to do more in the family business now that she had had time to think and re-evaluate her role as a mother. Rowena felt she had more financial stability and wanted to continue to work so she could now have holidays. Jane recognised that health and the way she had tried to live a healthy lifestyle would benefit her as she grew into old age. Susan had also altered her life both in her career and her relationships. She said:

I think, I think your thinking changes, and you get to a stage probably when you have got enough experience behind you and you can see enough in front of you to think, I have got to change things now and now I have actually got the courage to do it.

It seems too simplistic to explain this time of reflection and evaluation as solely the result of the end of reproduction. There was little reference to the freedom from worries about contraception or to the inconvenience of menstruation, and I have argued earlier that women who had finished with periods still identified themselves as menopausal at the age they had reached now. However, there was some indication from the narratives that the public expectation of menopause as a marker in the life-course of women gave them permission to pause and reflect in a way that was not available to men.

There was speculation about a male menopause and the way that men often appeared to react in an irrational way. The women gave examples of men behaving as though they were still young, feeling threatened by other younger men and the need to prove their sexual prowess. Many of these images fitted the middle-aged male stereotypes, but the women were able to talk about men they knew and whom they thought had experienced some crisis of confidence. Mary thought that men felt differently from women about growing older: 'I think it is different, yes. I am not sure whether it is more to do with their minds than their bodies.' The narratives of the women showed a degree of sympathy because men appeared to find it difficult to think about what age meant to them. Joyce had been talking about the popular view of middle-aged men and then offered a possible explanation:

> Probably they [men] view it different than us. But, then they haven't got the physical sign of, like we have got our periods, we have got flushes, they do have things like that are happening to them, but it isn't physical. I feel sorry for boys when they were going through puberty, because they haven't got a period for us to know that 'oh, she is going to have a period that is why she is feeling a bit ratty'. And you hear people who give an excuse for being so unsociable, whereas if it is a girl you say, 'oh they are going through their periods so that is okay'. But boys, they have got no physical sign, so you don't give them any leeway, do we? For men, probably we don't give them any more leeway because there is no physical sign, as I have said, and they do it on their own.

I am arguing here that the women perceived the ending of menstruation and, by implication, the end of their reproductive role around the expected age of 50 as a marker that gave them permission, both privately and publicly, to reflect and think about their lives and how they may shape them in the future. It could be said that changes in society's structures have removed many of men's scheduled mid-life transitions, such as retirement from paid work (Phillipson, 1998), in a way that is different for the current cohort of women.

Recognising the changing private self

Menopause has been recognised by some writers (Sheehy, 1994; Richards *et al.*, 1997) as a time of silent change, conducted in private unless there are noticeable problems, such as the requirement for medical intervention. The women who shared their experiences with me were aware that an inner change was taking place within themselves, which they acknowledged as happening recently: in their mid- to late forties. Ella was talking about the differences that she had noticed about herself recently:

> To be honest with you, I don't really know what it [menopause] is apart from putting it to age. So, if it is, if I am thinking about age, I am thinking, yes, perhaps I am. It is as if I have suddenly grown up. I think before, I think I was just going through the whatsit [menopause], but now I have more sense of direction, I am more focused.

Jenny too spoke about the age she had reached as giving her a greater awareness of how she fitted into the life-course: 'I think there is something about maturity, whatever that is. You get a bit of a perspective on it because you have been around longer and you see more things'.

Developing self-determination and self-definition

This realisation of menopause as a private change in the psychological development of women is supported in the research of Terri Apter (1995, 1996). She carried out a longitudinal study in the UK and the USA of eighty women who were aged between 40 and 55 years. She concluded that as they approach 50 the majority of women become more determined to resolve old conflicts and satisfy suppressed desires, and this was more to do with their time in the life-course than with the effects of a biological menopause. She explains:

> At mid-life women's development appears muted. It is far more private, and there are fewer players [compared with infants and adolescents]. Its silent but sure pace has led many people to believe that mid-life change is hormonal – another by-product of women's reproductive system. But psychology is a listening science, and in listening to women I could trace a deliberate acquisition of self-determination and self-definition – a matter of psyche, not biology.
>
> (Apter, 1995: 13)

I found this development of an inner self-assurance and self-determination to be present in all the women's narratives, to varying degrees, but it was most pronounced in the lives of women who had experienced other dimensions of oppression. Kathy spoke of the importance to her of reaching 50, when she felt she had finally grown up and no longer needed to be afraid of adults. She had been profoundly deaf since an illness when she was 2 years old and she told me:

> I am beginning to feel now I am an adult. Most of my life, particularly during my formative years, I was put down by adults, one man in particular, one teacher. I had to wear a big black hearing aid at school, with two great big black valve batteries, huge things. I was very, very overweight, I was ten at the time. He used to call me out in front of the class to hold my hearing aid out, with 48 class members to shout down it how to spell words I'd misspelt. So, I have always been put down by adults. It is true. I feel, just now this last month or so, hey I am an adult, why should I be frightened by other adults?

Jean had experienced racism since coming to Britain in the 1960s and she explained to me how her response to this had changed:

> The change is not so much that life gets serious but it is, you have lived it and you think, 'oh well', when you get a certain age. It's not that you don't want to fight any longer, you recognise what that fight is about…it is not about you and division, it is about everybody else. I suppose, because I mean, for me racism, I have had a fair amount of racism, but it isn't just me. It is the black community that racism is aimed at. Once upon a time, I would have probably wanted to knock their lights out. Now, I am thinking, 'Well, you are missing out. You are missing out on something, I can teach you. I know about you, you don't know about me'.

The women who participated in this study were able to articulate that they were experiencing inner changes of self-determination and self-realisation, which they linked to an understanding of maturity. However, this acceptance of mid-life change was also influenced by the external messages that come from the public sphere, which present negative images of older women's identities and their place in the social world.

Hiding from the public gaze

During the interviews, I was continually struck by the way in which the women made reference to other mid-life women, passing judgemental statements because they perceived them as being different from themselves.

Once my awareness of this was raised, I began to hear and feel it in my everyday experience, among my own friends and other women I observed. I realised that, by speaking of others, we were joining the public voice of ageism and were colluding with a social world that feels hostile to women as they pass their reproductive years. It seemed possible to construct an external self that was different from the maturing inner self, and that this process of maintaining a public image which was acceptable to others was a way of managing and accepting the realisation of becoming an older woman. There were various examples and strategies that the women adopted to pass as younger women, which included pleasure at being thought to be younger than their chronological years as well as examples of trying to look younger in appearance.

Passing as a younger woman

The concept of 'passing' has been documented in the feminist literature (Rich, 1984) and is a way that women can collude with the expectations of a patriarchal society. It has also been used in gerontological theories in the metaphors of 'masks' and 'masquerade', describing how people put on a mask to solicit a certain 'gaze', and pass themselves off in a false disguise (Woodward, 1991: 148). Many of the women demonstrated a reluctance to give their age to others or to admit to middle age. They took great pride in telling me stories of how people suggested that they were younger than their years. I asked Julia how she thought she was perceived by others, and she replied:

> I don't think they associate me as being as old as I am and I have had that throughout my life actually, you know, even just very recently. Going round people of 50 and they are saying to me, 'well of course when you are 50 you will...', 'well', I say, 'hang on a minute, you know, I am 50'. Or they will say, 'oh well, when you get up to my age', and they are 53 and you say, 'well I am not far behind you, anyway' and they have said, they don't take you as being that age, they take you as being in your middle 40s.

Julia had identified with the concept of self-assurance throughout the interview but was pleased to be considered younger than she was, which, I would suggest, was a reflection of the negative way that older women experience the social world. Claire told me about the remarks from her two children, who were in their late teens:

> I know my daughter always comments. When we go out on a Saturday night, she will say, you always look nice and you always, you know...I

wouldn't go out, it's not vanity. My son, he will say, 'one of my friends saw you' and say, 'oh, you look nice', so that makes you feel good. He said something about, one of his friends said he thought I looked young for my age, and I said 'that is a nice compliment but a kick in the teeth after'.

The women liked to pass themselves off as younger than their years; this helped them to maintain an identity with which they were familiar and comfortable at a time when they had been identifying changes within their own self-perception. They were aware of the emergence of new roles and a changed understanding of self-identity, but the reinforcement from others that they were still young was important in realising the similarities while the transition was taking place. Jenny was an exception to this general denial of age in the stories. She told me she loved describing herself as middle-aged and went on to explain:

Because I think it is the truth and I feel, I suppose it is a sort of resistance to the fact that people see it as not being a good thing. It is the fact that I am not a young person, I am not an old person, I am a middle-aged person, and I don't see that as derogatory. I don't like to be an honorary young person, I work a lot with younger people and you often hear people saying, 'oh, you are not a middle-aged person.' I say, 'yes I am, yes I am exactly like I am', and I worked hard to get like this. I didn't get fresh out the egg like this and I do think there is probably a period of your life that you are no longer, and you don't know from the starting point, you don't go, 'God I am 38, middle-aged I am 42', but I do think there is a point at which you are quite different. In some ways you never change, but there is a sense in which you are different to how you were when you were younger.

Jenny recognised that there was a negative image attached to being an older woman but she had integrated that into the greater understanding she had about herself, which she had gained through experiences in her life. She confirms that a transformation, of which ageing is the epitome (Andrews, 1999), does not have a clear beginning and end, but when there is the advantage of hindsight it is possible to see where the change occurred. Jenny had progressed to a stage of development when she was able to resist inclusion in the category of youth, which ultimately would be futile, because she had recognised that ageing is an inevitable part of the human condition.

No blue rinses and Crimplene dresses

The women also spoke of how they wanted to stay looking young and of how they wanted to be different from their mothers, whom they perceived as looking old at 50. They recognised that they belonged to a generational cohort and spoke of being 'baby boomers'. Sandra was acknowledging that she was reaching middle age and compared the difference with previous generations:

> Today I think women, and men I suppose as well, they make the most of themselves. They dress modern, they go out and they go on holiday and they have their hair done. Women years ago didn't do those things, did they? They [people in mid-life] dress modern, and have their hair done and have modern styles, I think it is great I do, I think it is lovely. I suppose we have got more money to spend on them things, than our mums and dads did.

Other women made reference to the horror of the blue rinses and Crimplene dresses that their mothers had had, and Rowena was clear that: 'I am not going to wear a beige anorak and a headscarf when I get older. I will wear bright colours'. They were concerned to live up to the previous images of their youth and were worried that society could apportion blame if they looked old or if they should, in one woman's words, 'let yourself go'. Helen expressed the views of many of the participating women in her response to our discussions on ageing:

> I feel that it is like something looming up at them [women] in perhaps the mid- to late 40s. We know that we are going to approach those years, and perhaps that is why we do battle again, trying to stay young, trying to look younger, we take more exercise. We are constantly thinking, 'how can I look better?', clothes, makeup, hairstyles. It is a battle and it gets worse as you get older, obviously.

Helen was highlighting the social realities of the public world and demonstrated the pressure to maintain that appearance of youth. A little later in the interview, she acknowledged her realisation of a changing more private identity when she said:

> When I think of the middle years, I think there are other qualities that should be emphasised. I am not saying that I want to be treated as a young girl, I don't. In fact, I used to resent being treated as a young girl when I was a young girl [laugh]. But it is finding this balance really, you don't want to be disregarded, 'oh she is old, she is frumpy'.

Women in this cohort have been exposed to images of young, thin, predominantly white women and to a fickle world of fashion which is aimed at youth. It has excluded women in different social and ethnic groups and those with diverse experiences of being a woman and it has challenged whether it is possible to maintain this image in a competitive world. The women in this study have argued that there is far more pressure on their generation to stay looking young than there was on their mothers, and they are trying to understand what that means for their lives. Ella, who was born in the Caribbean, raised a number of interesting points when talking about previous generations and ageing:

> Looking at the things, like the American thing, our cousins over there, because of this thing of, they have to be keeping fit, they have to be having the plastic surgery. I think perhaps in Britain, we are still a little bit away off, it is only certain people in this society, but I think it will go to the classes. I think it will be like the working-class person will see that as only a dream, whereas the middle class and the upper class, they will be trying to achieve this immortality a lot in time.

She then brought into the conversation, the dimension of race and ethnicity:

> I think that yes, black people again like anyone else, they want to look good and so on. But, I think because we have been a fortunate race in as much that we don't age as much as the Caucasian, I feel that there is no big problem about, if we age we tend to age more gracefully.

She identified that the pressure to stay young through plastic surgery was only an option available to people with higher incomes, and therefore excluded many women. She then joined the public debate in acknowledging the value of youth by comparing how fortunate black women were because they did not show their age to the same degree as their white sisters. Ella had been clear throughout the interview that she recognised a maturing of her inner self, but she joined the public arena when talking of the external self.

Conclusion

In this chapter, I have discussed how a group of women, aged between 45 and 50, with diverse and different biographies, gave meaning to menopause. They roundly rejected the biomedical model of menopause as a deficiency disease requiring treatment in order to prevent them becoming ill as they grew older. But, they did acknowledge that their bodies were changing by ceasing to menstruate. This, however, was understood in the context of 'being a woman' and as having an adult life experience of a hormonal cycle. Instead, the women spoke of menopause as a legitimate time, in their late forties, to reflect upon and consider themselves. It was a biological marker, a scheduled event, but one which gave them an opportunity to pause and reflect and which many of them recognised was not available in the same way to mid-life men.

This recognition of a maturing identity is in keeping with psychodynamic theories in which mid-life is considered to be a time when people become more self-assured (Erikson, 1982; Biggs, 1999a). What is less evident from the existing literature is how much that experience may differ for men and women. The women that I spoke to recognised their ageing identities, but hid them from the public gaze. They showed that at times they passed as younger people and joined the 'masquerade' (Woodward, 1991; Biggs, 1999b), adopting a public image that denied their ageing selves. They were aware too of the consumer pressure on them to stay young, and how that formed part of their shared history with others of the 'baby boomer' cohort. The 1960s have been talked about as prosperous times, when the youth culture was born (Featherstone and Hepworth, 1990), and the commercial world responded by developing a whole range of consumables for youth, which enabled the young to feel revered by society. It is this cohort which is now reaching mid-life and is particularly susceptible to the marketing of products which present an opportunity to stay young. Hormone replacement therapy is one example of a product which is marketed as a means of retaining the appearance of youth and defying the decrepit images of old women. The bent, little old woman with osteoporosis or the woman with dementia are powerful reminders to the 'forty somethings' of what old age may bring.

In conclusion, the outcomes from this small study, conducted within feminist and psychodynamic theoretical frameworks, have implications for how we perceive women at the menopause. It clearly suggests that the biomedical model is an inappropriate way to understand mid-life women. Instead, we need to recognise the changing inner identity that occurs at this time in the life-course. We need also to recognise and challenge the hostile social world that women encounter as they pass their reproductive years and to create and embrace new roles as women enter mid-life.

6 Older women undergraduates

Choices and challenges

Patsy Marshall

Introduction

Older women who enter higher education in order to study for a degree are challenging several myths. Among these are that older women should stay within their traditional roles; that older people are unable to learn; and that education is for the young. Some commentators have argued that older people should not be permitted to enter higher education:

> It is questionable whether a national educational system should be obliged to admit to its most expensive courses students who will never use their degrees or qualifications, or who can have very little time to do so.
>
> (Laslett, 1989: 167)

The counterargument that older women should become undergraduates is based on the notions of equity and social justice (Morwenna Griffiths, 1998). Furthermore, some educational gerontologists claim that the experience of undertaking education may empower older people (Glendenning and Battersby, 1990). However, empowering people is complex (Tout, 1995) and depends on the type of education (Percy, 1990; Glendenning and Percy, 1998) and how it is provided. What we do not know is whether older women are in fact empowered or disempowered through entering and experiencing higher education.

I was over the age of 50 when I first entered higher education and felt academically and socially anomalous in that setting. I had not anticipated being altered by the process, but found that inevitably I was changed. As an 'educational returner', feelings from previous schooling experiences were awakened. As a newly retired woman, I had to maintain a balance among the demands of higher education, my husband and family and pressures from those who thought I had 'time on my hands.' I wondered whether other older women university students had similar feelings and experiences.

Consequently, I decided to focus my doctoral study on women undertaking a first degree at the age of 50 plus.

The study was focused on three distinct educational phases and their repercussions in the lives of older women undergraduates. These three phases were:

- women's experiences of secondary schooling;
- the process of deciding to enter higher education;
- the experience of being an undergraduate.

Establishing a theoretical base for the work was complicated because a study of older women undergraduates fell across several disciplines, with a range of theoretical frameworks. The theories which informed my study came from two broad categories. In the first group were theories which emphasise the identity, individuality and diversity of the experiences of women as they age. Some, for example feminism and life-course theories, are outlined in the introduction to this book. However, also included in this group is continuity theory, which describes how individuals maintain their identity while at the same time experiencing change (Atchley, 1993).

The second group of theories related to the processes and outcomes of education. Here, I draw on social reproduction theory, which proposes that schools play a part in maintaining the status quo (Althusser, 1971, and Bowles and Gintis, 1976, cited in Madeleine MacDonald, 1980). Also included is cultural reproduction theory: the reproduction of the dominant culture via the school curriculum (Bourdieu, 1977) and the sense of moral order reproduced in schools which helps shape the culture of society (MacDonald, 1980). Cultural capital is apparently available to all but, in reality, is limited to those who have been endowed through their class and education to avail themselves of it (Bourdieu, 1977).

The low incidence of older women among undergraduate students in Britain has led to their being largely ignored by researchers. Additionally, as Kim Thomas (1990) notes, research about minority groups tends to stop at higher education as undergraduates are considered the 'fortunate few'. However, the quantitative study of older students by Stephanie Clennell *et al.* (1987) is useful in establishing the capacity of older students to learn. Also, two qualitative studies of mature female undergraduates help to provide a background to this research. Gillian Pascall and Roger Cox (1993) carried out semistructured interviews with forty-three women at two institutions of higher education in the early 1980s and 1990s. Rosalind Edwards (1993) studied thirty-one mature women social science degree students who were born between 1943 and 1966. A study of ninety-six younger students by Kim Thomas (1990) was also included in the literary base because its perspectives have resonance for older women undergraduates. Thomas (1990) was particularly interested in the origins and outcomes of why certain subjects at university attracted/repelled male/female students. Two government reports also provide background material. The Dearing Report (Dearing, 1997) on higher education, the first since the Robbins Report in 1962, provides a useful overview of higher education in the mid-1990s, whereas the response of the Secretary of State for Education and Employment, David Blunkett, incorporated in *The Learning Age* (Blunkett, 1998), highlights the Government's interest in adult education.

The study

My research targeted those studying at two campus universities, Keele and Luton, and those with the Open University (OU) living in the Keele and Luton catchment areas. I selected these universities because, while not claiming epistemological privilege (Jennifer Mason, 1996), I hoped to utilise having been an older female consumer of education in the OU and at Keele University. Also, living in the catchment area, I am a potential consumer of courses offered by the University of Luton.

The difficulties of identifying and contacting older women students are related to their low incidence and consequent low profile in university statistics. Campus university staff provided computer lists of women undergraduates aged 50 plus. Although initial contact with OU students was attempted via their tutors, this method proved less successful than approaching students via the OU area computers. Not all the students with whom I was put in contact were interviewed. In all, twenty-four women were interviewed: eight from Keele, seven from Luton and nine from the OU. They were a diverse group, and although they were at the same university or living in the same area none of them appeared to be in contact with anyone else in the study.

I adopted a qualitative research methodology to enable me to uncover the individuality and richness of the experiences of older women undergraduates, giving 'voice to the voiceless' (Sara Arber and Jay Ginn, 1995; West, 1996). I therefore tape-recorded a semistructured interview with each woman. Interviews varied from three-quarters of an hour to more than two and a half hours. They took place in universities, in the woman's home or in my home. I took a feminist approach to the interview process, placing the woman central to the narrative and not as an adjunct to her husband or family. Some women reported that this was the first time they had had the opportunity to tell and/or understand their story.

Defining the social class of women is complicated because it is dependent on male rather than female occupations and may change with marriage and other events in the life-course. However, of the twenty-four women interviewed, half could be considered to be middle class and half to be working class; half were married and about half were single or no longer married. Two of the women reported that they were menopausal. Two had considerable mobility problems, two were in very poor health and one was profoundly deaf. Only two black women were put in contact with me and one of these declined to take part. The choice of degree topics studied by the respondents lay more in the arts than in the sciences.

The findings

For this chapter, I have concentrated on how the three educational phases identified in the introduction to this chapter interacted with the women's senses of identity and how, or whether, they felt they had been changed by each experience.

Women's experiences of secondary schooling

They're going to get married and have children.

(Fiona)

The majority of children in the 1940s and 1950s (and into the 1960s) sat the eleven-plus examination in order to 'win' a place at grammar school. The results influenced not only their secondary schooling but also their sense of identity. What they did not comprehend at that time was that the examinations were culturally biased. Five of the seven women in this study who had to resit or who failed the examination came from working-class families. Some of those involved in the administration of the eleven-plus in the 1950s appreciated that the system worked against children from these families (Addison, 1985).

The eleven-plus was also gender biased. Boys were considered to be 'late developers' and eleven-plus results were weighted in their favour (Sutherland, 1984). Parkes (1986), writing about loss, connects the resolution of change and disruption in the life-course with subsequent sense of identity. One woman in my study, Edith, was still grieving for her loss of opportunities because she did not pass the eleven-plus. She discovered through subsequently studying sociology that the eleven-plus examination may not have been fair:

The tests were actually skewed because too many girls were passing and that made me angry. It could be one reason why I am doing my degree now.

Pauline's sense of identity was confirmed by her eleven-plus failure. She not only entered a less academic secondary school but also suffered a stigmatising comparison with a more successful older sister.

> My sister went to high school and I went to a secondary school... [so how did you feel about that?] Well pretty bad actually...I was always the pretty, practical one and she was the brainy one...

Whatever type of secondary school girls of these cohorts entered, feminists note that government educational policies, based on the belief that girls would become wives and mothers, ensured that their curriculum concentrated on homemaking pursuits (The Norwood Report, 1943, cited by Rosemary Deem, 1980; MacDonald, 1980). In the majority of grammar and secondary schools attended by the women in this study, mathematics and sciences were considered to be boys' topics, with girls often receiving less mathematics tuition and having their science limited to the domestic variety. As Irene recalled: '...girls weren't in those days supposed to be good at maths and like physics and chemistry...'

Many of today's older women were denied the cultural capital of knowledge of these subjects (Bourdieu, 1977). Poor mathematics skills can be devastating to the individual concerned (Hampshire, 1962, cited by Hajnal, 1972), and for some of the women in this study poor mathematics skills were reinforced by cruel teachers:

> She always insisted that you get a question right and if you got it wrong she used to cane you. The one thing I did learn was to lie, to cheat and be frightened for the rest of my life of figures.
>
> (Sue)

Because skills at mathematics and the sciences are frequently linked to intelligence, when skills in these topics become gendered, assumptions are made that boys (men) are better at mathematics and therefore more intelligent than girls (women). Ultimately, these perceptions affect the identity of women.

Some respondents who passed the eleven-plus were sufficiently changed and encouraged by their secondary education that they attempted to enter higher education. However, cultural reproductionist views of the proper outcome of the education of girls served to repress their ambitions. Kate's career plan was discouraged by her headmistress because it did not 'fit' the prescribed role:

> I wanted to do something different to teaching and she wanted all the

girls to go to teacher training college. I wanted to be a journalist. She told me that there were no women journalists. 'There's only one in the whole of Yorkshire' she said, 'and you should go to college and learn to be a junior school teacher, which is what all your friends will do.'

Parents also played a part in discouraging ambition in their daughters:

...[my] parents...thought 'oh girls it isn't important that they get educated because they're going to get married and have children. They're not going to need any education.'...I think that was it...

(Fiona)

Girls who had failed the eleven-plus and went to secondary modern schools had fewer options. Social reproduction theory was clearly in evidence when, before leaving their schools, Beatrice and Edith and their classmates were taken to local factories and shown the production lines, where it was presumed that they would work. However, Beatrice and Edith had been sufficiently changed by their schooling experiences, so they ensured that they worked in offices rather than in factories.

Deciding to enter higher education

But it's for me, first and foremost it's for me.

(Laura)

It is possible to identify at least three elements in the process of older women deciding to enter university. The first is how the decision was made; the second is the method of entry; and the third concerns the choice of university. Continuing education had not played any part in the adult lives of the majority of the women in this study. Many had been too busy raising a family and/or trying to earn a living with little or no academic qualifications. They did not have the time or finance to support any adult education. However, they did not consider studying for a degree after the age of 50 to be a discontinuity. Rather, for the majority, it represented a strong sense of continuity (Atchley, 1993), in that they were setting out to regain what they considered they had lost. As Zoë remarked, it was: '...to catch up with what you missed because you got married at twenty and you didn't have that chance did you?'

Some women only gradually appreciated that they wanted to enter higher education. Often, this occurred after they recognised that they had reached a time of transition in their life-course and that other changes were influencing their sense of identity. Gail, Zoë and Ursula had recently been widowed, although the husbands of Ursula and Zoë had previously divorced them. Six other women were undergoing or still feeling the effects of divorce or separation from their partners. Terri, for example, experienced a sense of freedom when her husband left her. By contrast, others became depressed or angry when their partner left. Zoë had spent years supporting her husband so that he could study for a degree. Then, he decided that he no longer needed her and she was devastated by the change in her circumstances. Some women had recently retired, and some felt that they had time on their hands after their children had left home. Others, by contrast, felt that they were suffering from too many demands and, as they aged, had difficulty in reconciling their own needs with their apparently compliant identity. After a lifetime's habit of putting the needs of others first, Yvonne spoke for many when she decided that she would give more priority to her own needs:

> …I had what I am sure is a fairly normal [reaction], …life is too short for me to spend time [on things] I don't want to do any more. You spend a lot of time saying yes I'll do this…or I'll go there and I thought 'no, I've had enough of this'. If I don't want to do it now, I am going to say I don't want to do that and use the time profitably doing things I want to do.

For others, the decision process to enter university was triggered almost casually when they went on an 'access' course, without fully comprehending that it was designed to enable mature students to enter higher education. Ros merely wanted to discover whether she could study at this level and found the work extremely difficult:

> I was terrified, absolutely terrified…I can remember spending a morning in tears saying I've got this essay to do and I don't know how to write an essay…I found it pretty traumatic and hard.

Others went on an access course to obtain qualifications for potential employers. However, because their tutors seemed interested in them and considered that they would be able to study at degree level, they were able to make an instantaneous and momentous decision to enter university. The decision thus became intimately bound up with the method of entry:

> We had only been there a few weeks when our tutor said well what university are you going to…we all looked at one another 'University? This wasn't on the agenda when we came'…and I thought well why not. If they think I've got the potential.

(Sue)

Like the tutors on access courses, friends or relatives also suggested to some of the women that they were capable of undertaking this level of study. The women who entered the OU were also influenced by OU advertisements. In general, they found that the OU system was efficient, and although some were not immediately able to enter their course of choice because it was oversubscribed they were kept informed and were supported throughout the admission process.

For a few of the women, the decision to enter university was much more planned. Although Laura had obtained an appropriate level of entry qualifications while at work, she decided that she would take early retirement, study for an A level and then enter a campus university. She had no extrinsic motivations for entering higher education:

> It's not an expectation to get a job. Also of course at my age…I am not thinking I must rush out to work. …But it's for me, first and foremost it's for me.

Laura's sense of identity, in particular being a black older woman and seemingly invisible to many white people, informed her decision to enter higher education. She did not intend to use her degree, but felt that knowing she had one would sustain and comfort her.

By contrast, many of the women had misconceptions about the possibility of their going to university: 'I tended to think you went to university straight from school' (Gail). Those who lacked self-confidence were diffident about applying for a place:

> …I really thought about it [going to university]. I didn't talk about it to anybody at all but thought about it for a couple of years and then still didn't tell anybody and applied because I thought well they won't have me.
>
> (Val)

Selection of university was informed by how much, or little, respondents wished the pattern of their lives to change. The majority made ease of access to their homes a priority. Two students, Ursula and Olive, took this to an extreme by obtaining campus accommodation. Of the thirteen other campus university students, six chose their university because it was easily accessible either by car or by public transport from their homes. Val selected her campus university and her study topics so that she could return home each day to lunch with her husband. Several women selected a campus university because they felt that they needed stimulus through interaction with other students and also with tutors. Some claimed that they were lazy and needed to be encouraged to work. They felt that OU courses would not meet this need. Another factor in selecting campus university study was that of time-scale. Campus university degree courses take 3–4 four years, whereas OU degrees, for those without previous degree-level qualifications, take a minimum of 6 years.

Some women also had a financial incentive for selecting a campus university over the OU. Before the abolition of student grants, as recommended by Lord Dearing (1997) and implemented by the Labour Government in 1998, first-time, full-time undergraduates of any age were entitled to a grant. OU study is considered to be part time, and part-time students were excluded from the grants system. Sue, however, experienced a major change in that she found that she was better off as a full-time student at a campus university than when she had been in employment.

For others, the OU appeared to offer flexibility. Irene and Gail selected the OU because they thought it would fit in with their work schedules. Fiona chose to study with the OU because she wanted to be free to select which course she would study. However, OU accessibility is complex. Although the OU's publicity focuses on study where and when you are able, in practice, after their foundation year course, students who wish to take part in tutorials with other students and tutors may have to travel considerable distances. The venues for tutorials are not known in advance as they are set up to give easy access to the members of any particular course. A student may therefore find that she lives in the centre of the group and does not have to travel far or that she lives on the periphery of the group and must travel some distance to get to tutorials.

A less positive reason for deciding to study with the OU is lack of knowledge about alternatives and a lack of confidence. Most of the women studying with the OU were unaware that campus universities would accept older undergraduates. Wendy's reasons for opting to study with the OU were related to her identity. She anticipated further educational failure and wished to protect herself:

> ...the thoughts that went through my head were, if I go public...I'm exposing myself if I can't do it or if I'm a fool or if I'm stupid, everybody can see... But if I do OU and I've got my own little study if I make a mess of it...it's only me that's sort of conscious of it...

Obtaining a degree in mid-life does not necessarily guarantee confidence in one's abilities or bring about changes in one's lifestyle. In the 1980s, Jane was aged 50 and thought that a degree in European history would improve her employment prospects. On completion of her degree she was unable to obtain a job in her topic and returned to secretarial work. When she retired in the 1990s, she decided to study for an MA at her local university. She went to the university with her husband to make an application but her plans were thwarted by the receptionist, who presumed that Jane required information about courses popular with older women.

> ...I said 'Have you got any information on postgraduate studies?' And she [the receptionist] said they were waiting for the brochure to be printed and they would send me one. So I said 'Fine' and we were just going then she said, 'Well would you like to look at last year's to get an idea?' so we said 'Yes'...we went and sat down and looked at it...[I] went back, gave it to her and...I said 'I can't find the post graduate'. And she said 'They do cooking and dressmaking at...[college]'. And my jaw just dropped. I was actually speechless...and my husband [said] 'It's postgraduate studies she said you know'.

Jane's lack of self-confidence meant that she did not pursue her goal. She decided that too many years had elapsed since her previous degree and that she would study full time for a second undergraduate degree.

The experience of being an undergraduate

> I always said if at any point [university] interfered with my family life then I would stop...
>
> (Yvonne)

Women aged 50 plus are very likely to have established their methods of coping with changes in their lives. This section therefore considers, first, how they incorporated the demands of undergraduate study into their existing lifestyles and, second, whether they felt changed, empowered or disempowered by their experiences at university. By entering higher education, older women challenge the norms about their proper behaviour (Gisela Labouvie-Vief, 1994), but, perhaps more importantly, some have accrued responsibilities that are not easily put aside. The potential strain upon existing relationships was pointed out to Sue at a campus university interview:

> Well I thought one [interviewer] was rather sexist...he said how did your family feel about your going into education. 'Are you getting support from your family?'...and he said 'well coming into education will either make or break your marriage' and it broke!

The women in this study had to find a balance between the demands of 'two greedy institutions' (Acker, 1980): their family and university. Edwards (1993), in her study of mature women undergraduates:

> ...identifies three main patterns of behaviour in relation to separating or connecting family and student life...women who strove to connect and integrate family and education; ...those who wanted to separate the two and lastly, those in the middle who connected some aspects but not all.

> (cited in Barbara Merrill, 1999: 12)

Like Edwards, I also found that the coping strategies adopted by the women to meet the private and public demands placed upon them were broadly in three groups, but that the groups were dynamic and fell along a continuum (see Figure 6.1). At one extreme were those who gave priority to a full-time caring role and ensured that being a student did not impinge on their partner/family, etc. I named this group the 'Caring Carols.' At the other extreme were those who gave priority to their studies. I named this group the 'Studious Stellas.' In the middle of the continuum were those who attempted to cope with public demands and private duties and felt frustrated and/or guilty about not being able to spend sufficient time on either. I named this group the 'Guilty Gerties'.

Perhaps because they have waited so long to enter university, 'Studious Stella' type behaviours predominated among the women. Three of the Keele students and two at the OU in the Keele area and three of the Luton students and one at the OU in the Luton area were 'Stellas.' In addition, two students at Keele, one at Luton and one at the OU in that area demonstrated more 'Stella' than 'Carol' type behaviours. Kate, who was divorced, exemplifies 'Stella' behaviour in that she determined to finish her studies in spite of her adult daughter's pleas for more attention:

> [What have you had to give up?] Nothing important. I mean the house was seriously neglected...My daughter towards the end, felt she did not have my attention when she had a lot of problems...she said 'Isn't our relationship more important than your studies?' and I didn't have

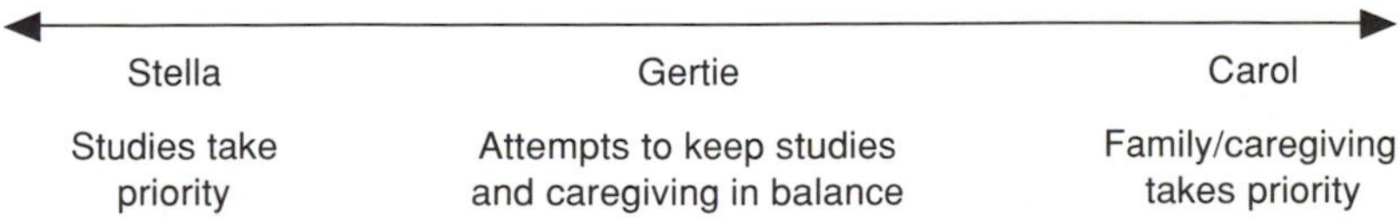

Stella	Gertie	Carol
Studies take priority	Attempts to keep studies and caregiving in balance	Family/caregiving takes priority

Figure 6.1 Dominant coping strategies continuum.

the heart to say 'no', but at the same time I thought I am not going to let go of the studies until it is finished…So I suppose I gave up putting my daughter first, but I didn't think that was a bad thing to do because she is 28 years old and that's her problem and not mine actually.

The husbands of 'Stellas' may have had to make some domestic or other adjustments. Pauline said of her husband, 'he has to work round me now'. Clare's husband seemed to have had other expectations of how she might spend her time, but Clare's wishes prevailed:

…my husband when I first started [thought]…I would have done better to get a job rather than studying …has been very supportive…

One student at Keele, two at the OU in the Keele area and one at Luton University demonstrated mainly 'Guilty Gertie' type behaviours. One student at Luton was more a 'Gertie' than a 'Stella' and one student at Luton and one at the OU in the Luton area were between 'Gertie' and 'Carol' in their behaviours. Women in the 'Guilty Gertie' segment of the continuum may discover that adding new roles and reviewing previous roles creates conflict. Ros felt guilt about her relationship with her daughter:

My daughter, I don't see as much of her as I would like to. And she's very supportive 'Oh Mum, I'm very proud of you'…but for me the old guilt's there certainly.

Beatrice found that managing housework and study was comparatively simple. Her difficulty lay in maintaining her studies while not impinging on the behaviour of her unemployed son:

…what I've found it's not so much finding the time to study, that's not the problem because there's nobody else. You juggle your things about to suit what you're doing. …No, that's not the problem. My son was the problem because he likes his loud music and the office upstairs is right next to his bedroom and no matter how much down he turns it you can still hear it…

One woman showed 'Gertie' type behaviour in endeavouring to cope with her studies and the demands on her time that had accrued since her retirement:

Well I've got more commitments now than I did then. 'Cos when you retire people think you have got so much time, 'Will you just do this?'…So I find that now my time is divided between quite a lot of things. I am spreading myself out a little bit thin and so I tend to not do things as well as I might do.

(Fiona)

Two students at Keele university and one at the OU in the Luton area had largely 'Caring Carol' type behaviours. 'Carols' endeavoured to ensure that those they cared for did not have their routine disturbed by the carer's studies. Val, as noted above, prioritised decades of companionship or habit above her studies. Another woman was careful to place her wish to go to university and her time spent in study in the context of their not having an impact upon the needs of her husband and children:

So I asked [her husband] if he minded…and I discussed it…with the children, that there will not be as much money but I would try as hard as I could that it actually did not make a lot of difference to them. And I have discussed it with them subsequently and they said 'no it hasn't' and they hadn't seemed to feel that the time that I have spent doing this has had a bad effect on them. But on the other hand I have always dropped everything even to doing my finals, when my daughter wanted an essay checking…because actually that's more important to me. …and I always said if at any point [university] interfered with my family life then I would stop.

(Yvonne)

Yvonne and Wendy, also at the 'Carol' end of the continuum, found time for study by regularly rising some hours earlier than other members of their households.

Study could also change how the women balanced the demands upon them. Maureen had previously demonstrated 'Carol' behaviour, but became more of a 'Stella.' As she put it:

I still am terribly bad at sitting down in my own home in my own garden because I…see the things that need doing. And once you start with the Open University, I could see the weeds grow and I could ignore them because I hadn't got time to pull them out. And I found this a strangely liberating experience.

Were the women changed, empowered or disempowered by their university experiences? Some university structures are inherently disempowering for all students. Lack of appropriate information about courses (Dearing, 1997) before and during the interview may lead campus university undergraduates to choose topics of study that they later regret. Older students who lack confidence when they encounter difficulty with their work typically do not seek help from tutors but place extra burdens on themselves. In an OU study, male and female undergraduates aged 60 plus were asked about their strategies for coping with falling behind in their work. Only 3% thought that they would contact their tutor, 14% decided to omit parts of the course and 40% made the decision to work harder (Clennell *et al.*, 1987). In my study, OU students who required personal support were reluctant to use the interactive part of the OU system and phone tutors at home because they empathised with the tutors and did not wish to disturb them. As Wendy recalled:

> ...I sometimes feel very much out on a limb. Although the tutors, there again it is my fault because I always see them as busy people, so to ring them up in the evening or a Saturday...I feel I shouldn't and yet there are times when I feel I could do with the help.

It is also possible to feel disempowered as an older woman because of lack of proper facilities. At Kate's campus university, young students waiting for tutorials sat on the floor in the corridor. Kate remained standing because she anticipated that she would look 'like a sort of stranded whale' if she tried to get up off the floor. Clare learned to avoid lectures where the overhead projections had been printed in a size 10 font. Yvonne felt that she was disempowered by her health problems, but did not expect any concessions from the university:

> I had a problem with the menopause...I couldn't remember anything....I went on HRT...and I was fine, but I still have a memory problem. In some ways you can't take it into consideration because you are all going for a particular goal so it's unfair to move the goal posts for some and not others.

Students with no previous adult educational experiences may feel further disempowered by having to sit examinations, and the problem may be exacerbated by having failed the eleven-plus. However, some women appreciated that the academic culture had changed their outlook:

> ...we hear of an article on the news and we are very quick to make a judgement, but now I can stand back from that...and think well superficially that looks as though that is the case but let's look at what's brought us to this situation. And so it's changed the way...yes it has changed the way I look at things...

(Ros)

Others had gained in confidence and widened their horizons as a result of their studies. Studying at degree level changed Irene's self-image:

> ...self doubt seems to be quite a common thing you do have. It [studying at degree level] gives you more confidence the further in that you get. You begin to think. I mean I would never have thought of doing a PhD before I started with the OU. That was something other people did...

Rather than feeling 'voiceless', as I had considered at the outset of this study, many women were in fact empowered by their university experiences. Some used their pre-existing skills in combination with the self-confidence that they had gained through study to improve the learning process for all students. Sue, a campus student, organised a meeting with faculty staff to promote changes in administration and courses. Several women also acted as intermediaries for lecturers who were unable to communicate effectively with students. Recognition from staff was also empowering, and some tutors discussed student/tutor issues with their older women students. Dee wrote to her Member of Parliament and to her Member of the European Parliament to ask for help in challenging the age limitations in the Student Loan Scheme and some women in the OU took the initiative in setting up support groups. Maureen felt so empowered, so changed, by her OU studies that for the first time in her life she went out to work. By contrast, Noreen felt disempowered and contemplated giving up her studies before obtaining a degree because her mobility problems prevented her getting to OU tutorials.

Conclusion: combating the myths

Why do a few older women defy myths about their roles and abilities by entering higher education? Activity theory suggests that the ageing self is likely to revisit activities previously found rewarding, but also that identity tolerates contradiction (Atchley, 1993). Continuity is evidenced by the determination of these women to study for the degree they feel that they were unfairly deprived of earlier in the life-course. The contradiction is that, although the majority had a negative experience of schooling, at a time of transition they seek the hazardous course of testing their abilities by returning to learning (Pascall and Cox, 1993). They may have found studying in university settings demanding, but there were compensations in discovering that educational methodologies had changed. Gail was able to compare her OU residential week experiences favourably with her memories of school days:

And one of the things that really...surprised me was the difference in the attitude between being tutors and students. It's so much easier now than when I was at school...You didn't chat to your teacher, you didn't even say 'Isn't it a nice day?' You said what you had to and that was it. Whereas you can exchange a joke with [a] tutor. ...At Summer School we were playing tricks on our tutors...

Although the majority of older women undergraduates are 'Studious Stellas' in that they give priority to their studies, their selection of university, particularly ease of access to home, indicates that they seek to fit their studies into their existing lifestyles. Terri, for example, selected a campus university because she thought she 'needed the discipline' but did not intend to alter her lifestyle to any great extent. 'I didn't see any point at the end of four years [in] having a degree and no friends'.

Once at university, the process of enlightenment through study undertaken later in life may be painful. Older students risk becoming more aware of the social injustices that they may have experienced in their lives (Griffiths, 1998). Their gender and previous lack of cultural capital had, for example, prevented them exercising influence and power in a hierarchical society:

It isn't until you realise their ideology and social construction and your upbringing and where you live, your environment, all these things that you never think about. You suddenly realise what a powerful effect they have on you...

(Wendy)

There is also the pain of discovering that study at degree level is difficult. The joy comes with the knowledge that, in spite of having previously accepted the myth that men are more intelligent than women, studying with men and women and with mature and young students confirms that intelligence is neither the prerogative of men nor are universities the preserve solely of young people.

These women, by completing courses and being awarded a degree, gain in confidence. Even Jane, nearing completion of her second degree, felt that she had been changed by the experience and was determined to implement her plans for her future. Where the women go next and what they do when they get there is open, but their university education informs their choice. For the majority of these women, their university experiences, particularly obtaining a degree, confirm their sense of well-being. At a time of transition in their life, they have moved forward rather than been thrown off course.

Universities should also recognise that older women are not just an older version of mature students. They have different strengths and needs. Their childhood educational backgrounds are different, as are their aspirations in studying for a degree. Not being career orientated, older women undergraduates are unlikely to contribute to the statistics about 'student outcomes' upon which universities have come to be judged. However, they have other contributions to make in higher education. They are able to give an honest opinion about how universities might be improved. They have time to appreciate and support the work of university staff. Lord Dearing (1997) stressed the need for universities to provide more work experience opportunities for their undergraduates. Older women undergraduates are able to contribute to this process by sharing their experiences of many years of paid and unpaid work with younger colleagues. Their biographies provide a warning that myths and stereotypes are likely to disadvantage older women. Their example reminds younger students that it is never too late for anyone to learn. Rather than wasting public resources as Laslett (1989) suggests, older women undergraduates enrich higher education. Universities should institute research to discover why the majority of older women do not wish to enter higher education. They should also be more welcoming to those few who do become undergraduates.

Note

Grants for undergraduates have now been replaced by the Student Loan Scheme for all students on higher education courses. Initially, people over the age of 50 were excluded from the Scheme. After some debate, the Secretary of State, David Blunkett, raised the upper age limit to 54 for those who intend to return to work (Carlton and Soulsby, 1999).

7 Women's voices in bereavement

Linda Machin

Introduction

Tradition, back to biblical times, has portrayed the widow as emotionally and socially vulnerable. Indeed, that vulnerability has been used symbolically to capture the worst of human losses. In more recent times, empirical research has identified the enormity of spousal loss as first in the hierarchy of human experiences of loss (Holmes and Rahe, 1967). The most frequent concomitant of widowhood is old age, and the two produce the double deficit of loss and stigma with grief and social marginalisation characterising the experience of older women (see Chapter 8). Early research into bereavement focused upon the widow (Marris, 1958; Parkes, 1972), but that emphasis has changed to include bereavement in childhood, loss of a child and parental loss (Beverley Raphael, 1984; Margaret Stroebe *et al.*, 1993; Klass *et al.*, 1996). This chapter looks at the changing theories of grief and women's place within it. It uses a current research project to illustrate the bereavement experience of women over the age of 45 (taken from a larger sample of bereaved people), in which the links among childhood attachment, adult attitudes to grief and the adult experience of bereavement are made. This study sample includes a range of losses, not just spousal, and represents a mix of women, from those carrying traditional female social roles to those whose experience and values have been shaped by the new possibilities in the post-modern world of the late twentieth century. The voices that speak offer contemporary insight into grief and those who experience it; they are heard both through the theories propounded by researchers and practitioners and through responses to the study which I have undertaken.

Women's voices in the theory of grief

The classic literature on bereavement was dominated by male researchers and theorists, while women, until recently, remained the subjects of that research. However, over the last three decades, women have entered the field as practitioners, researchers and grieving people using their own 'voice'. The perspectives which have arisen from this have been recognition of the diversity of expressions of grief and the normalisation of grief as a human experience. Key research and writing has come from Elisabeth Kübler-Ross (1970), Beverley Raphael (1984), Margaret Stroebe (1992) and Phyllis Silverman (1987) and from many unknown writers of single autobiographical accounts of their own bereavement experience. Unfortunately, the female contribution to the literature on bereavement is rarely acknowledged as separate from the overall literature on grief. However, by looking at some of the major women writers, it is possible to appraise their place in the development of concepts which have shaped new understandings about bereavement.

One of the first women to make an impact in the sphere of bereavement was Elisabeth Kübler-Ross (1970). She followed the practitioner/theorist tradition and used teaching seminars to consider the implications of terminal illness, both for the patient and their carers. Patients were invited to talk about their illness and the prospect of dying. This not only brought a new state of knowledge about terminal illness but also new recognition for the therapeutic benefits of talking about the experience. From this work developed a new awareness and confidence in addressing people's grief openly. Her work produced clearer definitions of the grieving process, building on the foundational work of Bowlby (1980). Commentators and students at times overlook the importance of these theoretical concepts by emphasising the apparent rigidity of the 'stages' notion of grieving (Kübler-Ross, 1970; Parkes, 1972; Bowlby, 1980). If one leaves aside the implied linear and sequential accounts of grief and if one understands them rather as descriptions of categories of experience, i.e. numbness, anger, guilt, depression, etc., they can be seen as characteristics which have an important place in any theoretical analysis of the bereavement experience.

The literature on bereavement is extensive and was characterised in the 1970s and 1980s by empirical and clinical studies aimed primarily at those people who are involved with supporting the bereaved. Beverley Raphael (1984) made a significant contribution to evolving knowledge in her book *The Anatomy of Bereavement*. By combining the existing, and new, theoretical knowledge with extensive case studies, she produced a definitive and systematic survey of bereavement. Her work was a comprehensive analysis of the human bonds which are broken by death: a life-course view of the experience of grief and a discussion about the circumstances of death and its consequences for the mourner. The work was intended to facilitate effective support of the bereaved by the caring professions. It characterised, therefore, a new era of macrotheoretical perspectives, embracing all categories of grief, not just widows, and translated the broader notions into practice principles.

Three new theoretical concepts concerning bereavement emerged in the 1990s. First, there was a move away from the dominance of the Freudian concept of 'grief work' as the singular psychological imperative when working with bereaved people. The idea of a *dual process* model of grief (Stroebe, 1992) suggests the importance of attending to restoration *from* grief as well as attending to the pain produced by it. Second has come a recognition that there is not an absolute end to the grieving process and the persistence of *continuing bonds* is not symptomatic of 'abnormal' grieving, as suggested by the classic theorists (Klass *et al.*, 1996). Third, there is now an emphasis upon the role of a *reconstructed biography* as a means of appraising relationships with the deceased and acquiring new existential equilibrium (Attig, 1996; Walter, 1996). These ideas do not reverse earlier theories, but offer explanations of grief and the process of managing it. They embrace a wider range of variants within the 'normal' and conceptualise the tasks within it as activities which are inherently part of the emotional, philosophical and spiritual routes to the restoration of balance and order. Women have played a role in this evolving process as leaders of new ideas (see, for example, Stroebe, 1992), as members of teams who collectively develop ideas (see, for example, Silverman, 1987) and as biographers/ autobiographers of their own stories and those of the deceased (Simone de Beauvoir, 1969; Marlena Frick, 1972; Harriet Sarnoff Schiff, 1977; Paula D'Arcy, 1979).

The 'dual process' model

Traditional theories of grief were grounded in the psychodynamic school of thought which conceptualised 'grief work' as an intense, introverted, emotion-focused activity. Anything less was regarded as pathological. Bowlby's (1980) theory of attachment, while following in the same tradition, began to broaden the concept of grief by understanding it as a social, as well as a psychological, phenomenon. However, the ideas about the way in which grief might be ameliorated were still based mainly on attention to feeling. Those people who are insecurely attached (Bowlby, 1980) and manage their grief by avoidance of feeling will be seen to demonstrate a pathological trait, termed 'prolonged absence of grief', and those whose insecurity generates an anxious symptomatology may demonstrate an alternative pathological trait, termed 'chronic grief'. These ideas have been firmly entrenched in the repertoire of the bereavement counsellor and used to create a systematic rationale for working with grieving people (Parkes and Weiss, 1983; Worden, 1991).

Margaret Stroebe (1992) has challenged the dominance of the emotion focus in counselling bereaved people. She and her fellow researchers have elaborated a model of grief in which there is a process of oscillation between rumination on painful emotions and attention to social adaptation to loss: a movement between 'loss orientation' and 'restoration orientation'. Diversion from feelings, which had previously been seen as avoidance and/or pathological, is now embraced within a broader definition of grief and viewed as part of the mechanism of adjustment. The implication of these ideas is very significant for practitioners. It gives the opportunity to see the different responses to grief as part of a spectrum of styles rather than a polarity between healthy and unhealthy, between normal and abnormal. It allows for what most practitioners have recognised, in a common-sense approach to their work, that social realities are hugely significant for people and play a part in emotional well-being too. It is important to distinguish the restorative (social) element of grief from the cultural messages of 'getting on with life'. The latter implies an isolated autonomy rather than the supported exploration of possibilities implicit in the Stroebe model.

This theory, although emerging from a team of researchers, has become especially identified with Margaret Stroebe. She has gone on to research the gender implications of the theory. She suggests that women, who have a greater social opportunity to discuss their feelings, tend to explore strategies for managing social change when they use bereavement counselling. Meanwhile, men, whose style of relating to others usually excludes attention to feeling, value that opportunity within a counselling context (Schut *et al.*, 1997).

The concept of 'continuing bonds'

Part of our traditional view of grief has been shaped by the medical concepts of illness and recovery. 'Getting over' a loss or 'coming to terms' with it are common ideas within our culture. Implicit in this view is the goal of separation from the deceased and moving on without her/him. Not to achieve this was thought to indicate pathology and a poor outcome. Practitioners, over the years, have observed situations in which persisting focus on the deceased has occurred, but in which, by any other measure of mental health, the bereaved person would not be deemed to be responding pathologically to their loss (Rosenblatt, 1996). Some important contemporary research has examined issues around the healthy resolution of bereavement and contributed to a redefinition of our understanding of grief. Klass *et al.* (1996: 355) describe this new perspective as:

> ...to shift [researchers and clinicians] focus from the end of the living bond to the place of the inner representation of the dead or absent person in the inner world of the survivor, and on the place of the inner representation in the survivor's social world.

This focus does not simply redefine the emotional response to loss, but embraces the wider meaning of relationships and life. This is more than a revisiting of memories: it is a fuller integration of the person of the deceased and the meanings held in the relationship with the deceased in the present and for the future. It could be argued that this is a perspective which has long been known to women and it is a notion incorporated within many cultures (Stroebe *et al.*, 1996). Only recently has a broader view come to challenge the male-dominated theoretical culture, which stresses the desirability of breaking bonds with the deceased. As research has moved to include qualitative as well as quantitative methods, so the individual voice of the grieving person is used to demonstrate these qualities of persisting connection with the deceased. A mother writes of the gentler 'older grief':

It's about sudden tears swept in by a strand of music...
It's about feeling his presence for an instant one day
while I'm dusting his room
It's about early pictures that invite me to fold him in
my arms again.

Older grief is about aching in gentler ways, rarer longing,
less engulfing fire.
Older grief is about searing pain wrought into tenderness.

(Klass, 1996: 211)

The concept of 'reconstructing biography'

If the *continuing bond* is a reconceptualisation of the ongoing nature of grief then one way in which the process of incorporation may be achieved is by the creation of a *reconstructed biography* of the deceased. Walter (1996: 7) describes the process as 'the construction of a durable biography that enables the living to integrate the memory of the dead into their on-going lives'.

Essentially, this is achieved through conversation with others who knew the deceased and can contribute to a joint construction of the biography. Walter regards natural social context as the most appropriate place for this process to occur and challenges the contemporary dominance of counselling as the primary source of therapeutic help. Attig (1996: 122) takes the idea further and looks at how reconstruction is a wider task of 'relearning the world' in bereavement:

When we grieve, we must relearn virtually every object, place, event, relationship with others, and aspect of ourselves that the lives of those who have died have touched. Our grieving takes as long as it does because there is so much to relearn.

While these ideas are largely being identified by male theorists, there is also a considerable body of biographical/autobiographical literature by bereaved people, many of whom are women (de Beauvoir, 1969; Frick *et al.*, 1972; Sarnoff Schiff, 1977; D'Arcy, 1979).

In sum, what do traditional and contemporary theories contribute to an understanding of women's experiences of grief and bereavement? Individually, they constitute a vast body of knowledge upon which practical treatment and caring has been based. Collectively, they affirm the complexity of grief as an experience and serve as a reminder that individual experience is as important a source of information about reactions to loss as are broader notions abstractly conceptualised as theories. For the individual bereaved person, making sense of experience is the macromanaging of microprocesses: it is coping with the emotional, physical, social, spiritual and intellectual consequences of loss by transforming the chaos into a newly meaningful order. Traditional theories have often been grounded mainly on the microprocesses, whereas contemporary ones are beginning to integrate these aspects of grief into larger units of meaning – units which do not dissect experience into unrecognisable components but allow the integrity of human experience to remain visible. The role of women in this process has often been as the subject of research rather than as contributors to knowledge within traditional theoretical frames. More recently, as diverse and less fixed perspectives emerge and there is a new emphasis upon qualitative research methods, the voice of women is being heard more clearly, as in my own research discussed below.

The experience of grief

Background to the current research

Some earlier research which I undertook (Linda Machin, 1980) together with my counselling practice pointed to considerable diversity in the way that people experience and give expression to their grief. As a counselling practitioner, it is crucial to recognise that wide ranging needs are a consequence of diversity within bereavement. Parkes and Weiss (1983) developed an 'index of bereavement risk' to predict those factors likely to contribute to a particular need for support in bereavement. The identification of variables likely to contribute to heightened vulnerability in bereavement does not account for all the responses that can occur. Some people experience a bereavement that was expected and timely, for example that of an older person after a period of health deterioration, but are overwhelmed by their grief, whereas, in other circumstances, someone might respond with equanimity to the death, for example, of a young person in an accident. What was becoming clear to me was the need to combine theories of grief, based on notions of universality, with a recognition that individual coping styles play a part in the range of reaction to loss. I was interested to see whether there is a pattern in the diversity by exploring what might contribute to an otherwise random manifestation of difference in bereavement. I began to set out these ideas within a framework, which I called the 'range of response to loss'. As a theoretical proposition, it seemed justified by both my research and practice experience. My current research attempts to establish the empirical justification for this framework.

The theoretical framework

I used the framework (see Table 7.1) in my bereavement counselling training repertoire as a way to help practitioners understand diversity in bereavement. In this context, it was affirmed by the personal and practice experience of counselling students. However, the questions still to be answered were: how useful is such a framework (a) as a theoretical description, (b) as a tool of assessment and (c) as an indication of which therapeutic approach might be most useful in counselling? Empirical examination of the hypotheses contained within the framework was called for, as well as reflection upon the connections with existing theoretical perspectives.

The framework begins by suggesting that early *messages* shape the child's concept of how loss and change are managed. These messages combine both direct verbal information which the child hears from parents and teachers and other messages transmitted culturally via the observable practices and behaviours of the people who inhabit the child's world together with other influences, e.g. the media. How these messages become internalised will depend upon the child's engagement with, and *experience* of, relationships and life events. The process of subsuming this dynamic of message and experience into an identity will result in *assumptions* about the nature of a person's own resourcefulness in the face of loss. A *response to loss*, therefore, is based on an acquired view of the world and 'my' place within it. This self-view will, in turn, produce a *response to other people's loss*; if loss is assumed to be overwhelming then not only am I caught within its pain but also I will have little energy for your losses. Conversely, if I see loss as controllable, I will urge upon you the same control which I exercise.

Collectively, this process of acquiring and interpreting experience fits with a number of theoretical propositions: Bowlby's (1980) 'internal working models', Parkes's (1993) 'assumptive world' and Marris's (1974, 1982)

Table 7.1 The 'range of response to loss' framework

	1	2	3
Message	Disabling	Enabling	Survival
Experience	Overwhelming	Accepted	Controlled
Assumption	I cannot deal with loss and change	I can face loss and change	I can control loss and change
Response to loss	Immobilisation	Use of own emotional resources and social support	Suppression or diversion from loss and change
Response to the loss experience of others	Minimise the significance of others' loss	Empathic response to others' loss	Pressure to suppress or divert from loss

Notes

Group 1 is characterised by a view of loss and change which is overwhelming; loss is emotionally and socially disruptive and the personal and social resources do not adequately mitigate against its immobilising impact. It is difficult to show appreciation of another's loss when overcome by one's own grief.

In contrast, *Group 3* seeks to control loss events and their affective consequences; emotional implications are minimised and coping strategies are maximised.

Group 2 is able to confront the negative and appraise the positive elements of loss in the knowledge of inner resourcefulness and external support.

'structure of meaning'. Each of these theories addresses the same processes which I am exploring in my proposed framework, i.e. that of the acquired sense of self, the world of experience and the responses which accompany that self-view. These theoretical perspectives also describe the structure and purpose of the process of making sense of experience; my framework articulates these structures and purposes. Furthermore, each theory, in some way, gains access to the working of those structures through the narratives that people use to describe experience, whether that narrative is the story told to the researcher or the therapist. Holmes (1993: 146) also asserts that: 'The narrative dimension in psychotherapy – helping patients to gain a clearer picture of their life and their early attachments – can be supported on scientific as well as aesthetic grounds'. Meanwhile, Mary Main (1991) has moved Bowlbian theory from an observation of attachment behaviours to a consideration of the place of narrative, in which the coherent quality of an adult autobiography is seen as a measure of attachment security (or insecurity). The psychodynamic paradigm (central to the development of theories of grief) is very different from the social constructionist paradigm, which holds that we come to understand ourselves in terms of the concepts embodied in language (Burr, 1995). However, the contemporary use of narrative in research brings the two perspectives into a parallel relationship with each other, if not into a theoretical synthesis. Both, therefore, have some place in offering insight into the data emerging from my study.

The study

My empirical study aims to look broadly at the characteristics of grief experienced by those people who seek counselling help in their bereavement. More specifically, empirical testing of the 'range of response to loss' framework was intended to examine the characteristics of the varied reactions to bereavement and sought to determine whether three categories could be identified. Verification of the framework would have implications for the practice of bereavement counselling; counsellors would be able to modify their approach to client work on the basis of the varied perceptions and coping styles brought by their clients.

The major theoretical perspective used to examine the framework was 'attachment theory' (Bowlby, 1980). Attachment theory helps to link this piece of research, on loss and bereavement, with other research in the last two decades (Parkes, 1991, Stroebe, 1992). In addition, a new measure has been devised to explore the connection between attitudes and grieving styles; attitudes result from the cognitive integration of internalised messages combined with experience. The research hypothesis is that they become indicators of how people react to events of loss in their lives.

This study used as its sample adult clients who had received bereavement counselling at Bereavement Care, a counselling service in North Staffordshire. Clients were invited to participate after their initial counselling session. The distance from the death of their relative/friend was variable, but it was at a time when they were identifying, within themselves, a need for some help with their grief. The research process was carried out quite separately from the counselling. An appointment was made for a research assistant to visit the client in their home to facilitate the completion of a three-part questionnaire. Respondents were invited to participate in the research on a second occasion, 6 months after the first interview, to complete the third part of the questionnaire again.

Part 1 of the questionnaire included an account of relationships, experiences of loss and change and a subjective reflection on the emotional characteristics of childhood (before 16 years old). Part 2 of the questionnaire invited a reflection upon adult perceptions and experiences relating to relationships, loss and change. Part 3 included standardised psychometric tests, such as the Beck Depression Inventory and the Impact of Events Scale, and questions focusing upon the social and emotional circumstances after the respondent's current bereavement.

Empirical testing of 'response to loss' categories, as set out in the theoretical framework (see Table 7.1), was undertaken by designing a new measure of 'self' perception in relation to grief. The measure was called the 'adult attitudes to grief'. The 'attitudinal' measure was devised and piloted using a sample group of university students. The resulting nine attitudinal statements, which exemplify three attitudes within each of the three categories in the framework, were then used in the main study (see Table 7.2). Responses to the statements were made on a five-point Likert scale, ranging from 'strongly agree' to 'strongly disagree'.

The three categories in the framework were justified by statistical analysis of the responses to the 'adult attitudes to grief' scale, using the Cronbach Alpha test. Having justified the three styles of 'response to grief', the data were used to examine, more fully, the social and psychological characteristics associated with each of the categories.

Mid-life and older women's responses to loss

Thirty-nine women over the age of 45 years were interviewed at the first stage of the research and thirty of these remained within the study for the second interview. Their ages ranged from 45 to 80 plus; nine women were

Table 7.2 The 'adult attitudes to grief' scale

The following attitude statements exemplify group 1: 'overwhelmed' in the framework

1   For me, it is difficult to switch off thoughts about the person I have lost
2   I feel that I will always carry the pain of grief with me
3   I believe that nothing will ever be the same after an important loss

The following attitude statements exemplify group 2: 'accepting' in the framework

1   I feel able to face the pain which comes with loss
2   I feel very aware of my inner strength when faced with grief
3   It may not always feel like it, but I do come through the experience of grief

The following attitude statements exemplify group 3: 'controlled' in the framework

1   I believe that I must be brave in the face of loss
2   For me, it is important to keep my grief under control
3   I think it is best just to get on with life after a loss

---

in the forties age group, thirteen in the fifties group, twelve in the sixties and five were over 70 years of age. Twenty-one women over the age of 45 had suffered the death of a spouse or partner, five were the adult child of the deceased, four had lost a child, six a sibling and the remaining three had sought counselling help after the death of a friend.

For those women seen twice (where it was possible, therefore, to have a picture of counselling over a period of time), the amount of counselling varied from one session to more than twenty, the average for the sample being 7.6 sessions. Although the study did not primarily assess the efficacy of counselling, it was a factor to be recognised as part of the support system which had been initiated by the respondent.

When looking specifically at responses to the 'adult attitudes to grief' scale, as an indicator of the style of coping with loss, at the first interview twenty-two of the thirty-nine women (or 56%) were 'overwhelmed' in their bereavement, i.e. came within group 1 of the framework. At the second interview, twenty-one of the thirty women (or 70%) fell within this category. This apparent increase could be accounted for because those women who were still having a need for counselling or other support in their bereavement were more likely to stay in the research than those who felt that they had moved on.

The women 'controlling' their grief response, i.e. those associated with group 3 in the theoretical framework, totalled seven at the first interview and four at the second. Within this sample, it is probable that those women who managed their bereavement by having a controlling response to it were less likely to use a counselling service.

Five women had an equal scoring between groups 1 and 3 ('overwhelmed' and 'controlled') at the first interview and group 3 at the second interview. This seems to be a qualitatively different response to bereavement from the 'accepting/balanced' perspective of group 2 in the framework; it seems to be less the process of healthy oscillation between loss and restoration orientation (Stroebe, 1992) and more a tension between being 'overwhelmed' and being in 'control'.

Only two women scored in the 'accepting/balanced' category at the first interview, and one woman at the second interview. Two further women at the first interview had a combined score with this category and one of the others. At the second interview, three women combined their response of 'accepting/balanced' with 'control'. It is clear that, although there is overall statistical justification for the framework, some individuals span more than one category, which is what might be expected when looking at the variability of individual responses.

Using the Leiden detachment questionnaire (Cleiren, 1991), thirty-five women in the sample felt that accepting their loss was very difficult. Of those who remained in the study (thirty women) at the second interview, all felt that accepting the loss was difficult. Within this measure, twenty-nine women 'longed for the deceased' and nineteen had difficulty detaching feelings from the deceased. Of those at the second interview who still had difficulty in detaching, seven of the nine were widows. In looking at the felt need for emotional support, expressed in terms of 'Do you have need to have someone put an arm around your shoulder?', of the fourteen who said that they had a great need, twelve were widows. When asked 'Do you have the feeling of being part of intimate social relationships?' at the first interview, twenty-eight women felt themselves to be to some extent or strongly part of such relationships. At the second interview, there was an increase in the proportion of women feeling outside intimate social relationships to more than half of the sample. Clearly, in the early days of bereavement, or at the time when people have an overt need for support, close relationships play a part. But, in this study, the stability of such support is not demonstrated over a period of time.

By way of contrast, when asked about the 'opportunity to freely express thoughts and feelings to others', there was a tendency for this to increase over time. Those who felt a persisting insufficiency in this dimension were in the 'overwhelmed' category of the framework and tended to have more counselling sessions. The opportunity to talk about the deceased declined over time, especially for non-widows in the sample, i.e. the need for widows to talk about their partner is more readily understood by other people. The memories which people wanted to share in their bereavement included events within the life of the deceased, the nature of the relationship with the deceased, the nature of shared experience and what the deceased had meant to other people.

Interviewers were asked to appraise the ease or difficulty of facilitating the completion of the questionnaire. About one-third of the women found the interview difficult or very difficult. This was most often because of the pain that was associated with the memories and experiences they were sharing. For some, it was difficult for them to remember details from their childhood. Others had difficulty in articulating feelings and experiences from the past. Main (1991) suggests, in her exploration of people's early attachment experience, that inarticulacy in describing early relationships and events is an indication of insecure attachment in childhood.

The presentation of data so far has provided information derived directly from quantitative analysis of the study material. However, the exploration of the material on an individual case basis also allows for more qualitative descriptions of respondents to be made; not only are there quantitative responses to the questionnaire but supplementary qualitative responses too. Using this method of individual scrutiny of questionnaires, three case studies have been chosen to explore the profile of the three different coping styles within the theoretical framework. Pseudonyms have been used to protect the identity of the women.

Women's coping styles

Alice was a 51-year-old widow whose husband had died suddenly of a heart attack. She sought counselling help within a month of his death. Her style of coping, as indicated by the 'adult attitudes to grief' scale, showed that she was 'overwhelmed' at both the first and second interviews, i.e. she was most closely associated with group 1 in the theoretical framework.

Alice was the only child of parents who divorced when she was a teenager, leaving her with her father. The messages from childhood (taken from items in the questionnaire) with which Alice could most easily associate were 'You have to get on with life without depending on other people' and 'People don't understand how difficult things are in our situation'. Childhood experiences, which were very difficult for Alice, were separation from her mother and her parents' difficult relationship. Additionally, the death of her grandfather and the suicide of an aunt were especially problematic for her. Feelings which characterised Alice's childhood were biased towards negative emotions, for example sadness, anxiety, depression and confusion, but included the sense that she was a loving and affectionate little girl.

As an adult, experiences of unexpected death were very difficult, as were problems in relationships and physical illness. Responses to the Impact of Events Scale showed that Alice was extremely troubled by intrusive thoughts and feelings about her dead husband. Her level of depression reduced between the first and second interview, but remained moderately severe. Alice found it very difficult to detach her thoughts and grief about her husband. While Alice had a great need to express thoughts and feelings about her grief, she felt only partially socially integrated at the first interview and not at all integrated at the second interview. The readjustments which she was having to make were a reminder that '…he made all the decisions. I find it frightening to make decisions and the emptiness is terrible'.

The interviewer reported that Alice chose to tell the 'story' of her husband's death before responding to the questionnaire. She was frequently tearful and, although she found the research interview painful, she expressed a sense of relief from having an opportunity to talk about her bereavement. Alice had made extensive use of the counselling service and, additionally, was receiving psychiatric help.

In summary, the emotional disturbances within Alice's childhood seemed to produce a fearful approach to life in which experiences of loss, change and bereavement produced particular vulnerability. This was expressed in a persisting sense of being 'overwhelmed' (group 1 in the framework) and in limited personal and social resources for addressing her grieving needs.

Barbara was aged 56 and had had ten counselling sessions after the death of her brother from cancer. Although there was an attempt to 'control' her feelings at the time of the first interview, this was set within a coping style of 'acceptance/balance', i.e. group 2 of the theoretical framework.

As a child, Barbara experienced some separation from her family as a result of a number of episodes of illness which took her into hospital. This produced a particular difficulty associated with medical procedures, but seemed to put many of the other experiences of loss and change in her childhood into perspective. Barbara associated her childhood with a spectrum of emotions – positive (happy, affectionate, trusting, loving, energetic) and negative (anxious, fearful, timid, bossy).

As an adult, Barbara found conflict in important relationships very difficult and, also, she had some difficult bereavement experiences. Barbara's sense of self within her adult relationships was characterised by finding it easy to be close to other people without carrying any anxiety about rejection by others or a fear of being hurt by them. Although Barbara was slightly depressed at the first interview, she was not depressed at the second interview. However, some intrusive thoughts and feelings persisted to the second interview. There was some ambivalence in the relationship with her brother, but the longing for him was very strong. While there was adequate opportunity for Barbara to share her memories with other family members, there was not the same opportunity for her to express her own inner thoughts and feelings about her brother. Counselling had become the place where these things could be shared.

The interviewer reported that Barbara had been an 'easy' respondent who had clear insights into her own experiences and, although these had been painful, she had inner strengths and was able to use external support (partly counselling and partly friends) to address her grief.

In summary, Barbara had acquired, during her life, strategies to deal with difficult situations; life had not been easy for her, but she had developed the capacity to recognise her own strengths within situations as well as the challenges which they produced. She used counselling when her own network of support was not adequate but, overall, was able to maintain a coping style consistent with group 2 of the theoretical framework, i.e. 'accepting/balanced'.

Carrie was 63 years old and her husband had died of lung cancer after a short illness. She had five counselling sessions. At both research interviews, Carrie demonstrated a 'controlling' style of coping with her bereavement, i.e. characteristic of group 3 in the theoretical framework.

Carrie was the youngest of four children. Her mother had died when

Carrie was 13, but she felt '...mothered by my sisters'. A message from her childhood (selected from the questionnaire) which typified what she heard as a child was 'it may be hard but there will always be someone to help you'. Carrie's reflections upon the feelings of childhood indicate that positive rather than negative emotions were dominant in her experience.

Carrie was moderately/severely depressed at both interviews and the Impact of Events Scale showed that she tended towards an avoidance of thoughts and situations associated with her grief. As an adult, Carrie felt secure in close relationships and had a stable conflict-free relationship with her husband. She felt strongly loved and valued within her social relationships but, nevertheless, felt that the support was insufficient for her to talk about thoughts, feelings and memories of her husband. Cards and messages of condolence from professionals such as the radiotherapist and the funeral director were particularly comforting to Carrie.

The interview was easy and was characterised by Carrie's resolve to build a new life. She was arranging to do some voluntary work and had made a new friend with whom she was arranging a holiday.

In summary, Carrie had experienced some difficult losses in her life. While her social network afforded a measure of support, it was insufficient to meet her grieving needs. One might speculate that Carrie had assimilated a dominant sense of 'getting on with life' and 'taking control'. This being so, she made use of counselling as part of a strategy to manage her bereavement and, after a short series of sessions, reverted to her own coping mechanisms. She demonstrated, at both interviews, a style consistent with group 3 of the theoretical framework.

Discussion

In each of the case studies chosen to exemplify the three groups within the framework, the women had suffered some disruption in their early years: parental discord, illness and bereavement. However, in spite of this, they each developed different styles of coping with loss. The contrasting styles, it seems, were not so much a factor produced by qualitatively different life events, but were related more to the way in which each developed a sense of self and made sense of their own experience. The recalled emotional characteristics of childhood give a distinctive sense of the three women and their life perspective. Alice's feelings were biased towards the negative, Carrie's were positive, while Barbara experienced a wide spectrum of emotions. This would fit with the expectation that a person overwhelmed by experience (group 1) is likely to be most conscious of bad feelings, whereas someone seeking to be controlling in their response (group 3) will focus on good feelings. The person who is accepting and balanced in their response to life events (group 2) is more able to acknowledge a range of emotions which span pleasurable and painful affect.

Distress, as measured by the 'impact of events scale', also shows characteristics which are consistent with the pattern articulated in the theoretical framework: Alice was troubled with intrusive thoughts and feelings, whereas Carrie tended towards an avoidance of thoughts and feelings associated with her grief.

In some way, all three women found limitations in their social networks. For Alice, her sense of social integration was not sustained over time, and one wonders whether her great need to express her grief was making excessive demands upon her social network. Barbara was able to share memories with other people, but her personally felt grief could not be expressed within her family and friendship circle. This might be that a sibling, in common wisdom, ranks as a lesser loss than, for example, a partner or a child. Carrie presents a picture of secure and loving relationships but, in spite of this, found that the support did not permit her to talk about the impact of her husband's death and its meaning to her. One might speculate that if she tended towards an avoidance of reminders of her grief, family and friends might use this as a cue not to speak about the bereavement.

The three case studies provide material that suggests that there are identifiable characteristics associated with the three groups in the theoretical framework. What seems clear is that these women do not fit within a particular category simply on the basis of their life experiences, but that a much more complex process of understanding the world and one's place in it produces the varied responses to loss. More generally, the study shows that women have a wide range of reactions to bereavement, most of which can be regarded as non-pathological. The relationships which are lost in bereavement all produce a grief, which needs to be recognised and understood: the widow, the bereaved mother, the bereaved daughter, the bereaved friend – all may seek, and deserve, support in the loss which they have suffered. This wide ranging population is appropriately the client group of a bereavement counselling agency.

Conclusion

The research described in this chapter has been influenced by traditional psychodynamic and psychological concepts. The theoretical framework used to identify the range of response to loss makes use of these traditional theories (Bowlby, 1980), but also reflects more contemporary thinking about the ways in which people grieve (Stroebe, 1992). Women have entered the field not only as the focus of men's research but also as researchers and theorists in their own right. Mary Main (1991) and Kim Bartholomew (1990) have continued the work of Bowlby by developing the theories of childhood attachment into an exploration of the significance of attachment for adults. Elisabeth Kübler-Ross (1970) has articulated the theory of grief in practitioner contexts. Beverley Raphael (1984) has broadened the scope of definitions of bereavement to include all categories and circumstances of loss. Margaret Stroebe (1992) has widened the concept of grief work to include attention to restoration from grief. Silverman and Klass (1996) have challenged the notion of letting go, implicit in traditional 'grief work', and replaced it with the concept of a persisting bond with the deceased: a relocation and reformulation of the meaning of relationship.

Much additional literature exists in the form of autobiography and biography in which stories of loss and grief identify the individual experience and response to bereavement. Theorists and researchers in many fields now see narrative, and the 'story', as an important entrée into the world of human experience (Holmes, 1993; Burr, 1995). Practitioners know that it is also the therapeutic route to self-discovery and meaning making for individuals. Such a shift in perspective has resulted in a new emphasis being given to qualitative research.

In this chapter, the voices of women have been heard both through contemporary theorists and bereaved women themselves. In my study, the patterns which emerged were ones which encourage us to look for diversity in expressions of grief and the need to be vigilant in our listening to each bereaved voice. It is the role of the counsellor to hear the voice, in both listening for the clues to styles of coping which may come from the attitudes towards loss and change and recognising the individual manifestation of grief. If 'attachment' theory is taken as a therapeutic indicator then it is possible to see that counselling should be a process attempting to create (or recreate) a secure 'attachment' for the client (Holmes, 1993; Marrone, 1998). The 'range of response to loss' framework suggests that optimal functioning may be promoted in which she can appraise the positive and confront the negative in her loss situation, while engaging with appropriate support.

Whatever the future direction of the study of women and their management of the transitions of mid- and later life, it seems certain that women will continue to have a central role as researchers and that they will be increasingly directing their attention to the voices and experiences of their sisters.

8   Widowhood in later life

Pat Chambers

Introduction

A review of the literature on later life tells us that widowhood is a women's issue. Although the age of widowhood varies greatly, it is primarily experienced by older women – this is because of gender differences in mortality and the social norm that women marry men older than themselves. The average age of widowhood varies according to class and race: the middle classes experience widowhood at an older age than the working classes; blacks experience widowhood at a younger age than whites (Markides, 1989, cited in Sara Arber and Jay Ginn, 1991). In Great Britain in 1995, 32% of women aged 65–74 were widows compared with 10% of men (OPCS, 1995). Widowhood therefore is the *likely* circumstance of older women and it becomes the norm as they move into old, old age. Among women who were over 75 years of age in Great Britain in 1995, the proportion of widows was 65% (OPCS, 1995), with an even greater proportion in the group who were over 85. Population projections suggest that the number of older people over 75 is likely to double by the middle of the twenty-first century (Age Concern, 1998). In subsequent cohorts, therefore, if current mortality rates continue, we are likely to see even more older widows.

Given that widowhood is such a major feature of later life, it is surprising to discover that research on the lives of older widows is so scarce. This is particularly so in Great Britain – the little research there is concentrates on loss and bereavement (Marris, 1958; Margaret Torrie, 1975; Ann Bowling and Ann Cartwright, 1982). Kate Davidson's (1999) work on gender differences in widowhood is one exception. North American research is more abundant (Helena Lopata 1973, 1987; Arling, 1976; Elizabeth Bankoff, 1983; Ferraro, 1984; Morgan, 1989); however, until the last decade (Ann Martin-Matthews, 1991; Eileen Jones-Porter, 1994; Lopata, 1996), there was still a concentration on loss and bereavement which presented a problematic if not pathological model of widowhood, as Mary Adlersberg and Sally Thorne (1992: 9) confirm:

The vast quantity of literature on older widows in our society convincingly portrays widowhood as an experience fraught with poverty, ill-health, loneliness, grief and readjustment.

My own curiosity about later life widowhood stemmed originally from a growing awareness of the differences that I encountered between the older widows I met in my own neighbourhood or in the course of my work and what I was reading in the literature. Many of these women, after a period of bereavement, appeared to be leading fulfilled lives and were certainly engaged in society in a variety of ways. I was so struck by the diversity of their experiences that I wanted to know more about what it was like to be an older widow and what had affected that experience. I wanted to try as far as possible to gain an insider's view of their world and add their 'voice' to the literature. A qualitative, biographical approach, which used unstructured interviews, seemed an appropriate way of enabling women to speak out about their lives. By focusing on the past as well as the present, it is possible to see widowhood as another passage in the lives of women and to explore the continuities and discontinuities that they bring to this time of their lives. Underpinning this quest is a feminist perspective and practice which aims to both understand and engage with the social reality experienced by older women of different ages, classes, races and disabilities (Shulamit Reinharz, 1992). This chapter charts my journey of exploration into the world of older widows in a number of ways:

- by reviewing the literature on later life widowhood and identifying prevailing myths;
- by exploring a variety of theoretical perspectives and considering their usefulness in understanding the lives of older widows;
- by considering an alternative approach to the study of later life widowhood;
- by focusing on the diverse experience of later life widowhood via the voices of a group of older widows participating in my current doctoral research;
- by challenging the stereotype of older widows.

Reviewing the literature

Much of the research on later life widowhood in the 1970s and 1980s was quantitative, conducted through the use of extensive questionnaires or structured interviews (Pihlblad and Adams, 1972; Lopata, 1973, 1987; Atchley, 1975; Arling, 1976; Bowling and Cartwright, 1982; Bankoff, 1983; Shirley O'Bryant, 1988; Babchuk and Anderson, 1989; Pat Sable, 1989;

Rosik, 1989). The focus of the research was on the problems of widowhood and the support systems available for older widows. The timing of the research in relation to widowhood seems to be crucial; both the American and the British studies were conducted within 3 years of the death of a spouse. I have suggested elsewhere (Pat Chambers, 1994) that, for some women, this could be seen as falling within the period they identify as 'bereavement' rather than their ongoing and developing life as a widow. Therefore, much of the literature on widowhood in the 1980s would be better construed as literature on 'widows in bereavement'. While the findings from all the research vary, often because of the different methods used, the overall picture of the lives of older widows is a fairly uniform one and has led to the development of a popular 'mythology' surrounding later life widowhood. These myths include:

* older widows are a homogeneous group;
* widowhood is synonymous with the acute state of bereavement;
* widowhood is an experience isolated from the rest of women's lives;
* older widows are not self-determining;
* older widows are lonely and isolated;
* widowhood is a period of decline.

As Helena Lopata (1996: 5) reminds us, the problem with myths is their stereotypical nature. Hunter and Sundel (1989: 21) suggest: 'Myths are dangerous when they result in oversimplified stereotypes that influence personal perceptions, social interaction and social policy.' Helena Lopata (1996) goes on to say that the interesting aspect of myths about widows (and widowers) in American society in the 1990s is their heterogeneous, sometimes contradictory, nature. This may be something to do with the fact that in current American (and British) society there are no longer any formal rules for behaviour in widowhood; the experience may instead be shaped by this contradictory mythology. Lieberman (1994, cited in Lopata, 1996: 6) develops this further:

> Widows are probably one of the most misunderstood groups in America today. As pernicious as they are pervasive, the myths about widowhood are far more harmful than its realities.

He further suggests that psychiatry and its practitioners have reinforced this problem model by viewing widowhood as a disease which needs either therapy or tranquillisers for recovery. Mary Adlersberg and Sally Thorne (1992) were initially influenced by this pathological model in their project, which sought to find ways of helping older widows to 'recover'. They found instead that their preconceptions were challenged by many of the older women who were referred to them, who saw widowhood as a time of opportunity. These women also reported that the myths of widowhood got in the way of them openly expressing these views to their families and friends who had believed the myths. In addition, the women themselves had internalised the myths and consequently felt guilty at reporting satisfaction and growth.

More recent qualitative research (Adlersberg and Thorne, 1992; Martin-Matthews, 1992; Susan Pickard, 1994) has started to question some of the prevailing myths of widowhood. Indeed, Lopata, who has written for 26 years on widowhood, now challenges some of her own earlier assumptions (Lopata, 1996). Widowed in 1994, she now writes from the perspective of a widow. Referring to the numerous myths, stereotypes and assumptions surrounding widowhood, she says:

> Even I found myself influenced by these at the start of the research. Many of these myths present a dismal and limiting picture of women.
>
> (Lopata, 1996: xiii)

Theoretical perspectives

Some of the theoretical perspectives used in the study of later life widowhood have served to reinforce the problem model and thus perpetuate the mythology. Role theory, particularly a decremental model of role loss, is the theoretical framework for a number of major studies on widowhood (Elaine Cumming and William Henry, 1961; Zena Blau, 1973; Lopata, 1973, 1987). There is some suggestion in the literature of a crisis for older women when they lose the role of wife. Lopata's (1973) work looked at the changing roles of widows in their adaptation to their new life and how for some women this proved to very difficult. Zena Blau (1973: 13) saw widowhood as a 'role less status', lacking any culturally prescribed rights and duties towards others in the social system. Ferraro (1984), however, identified some changes within family roles in the early stages of widowhood, particularly between mothers and daughters when the daughter might take on the 'mothering' role for a period of time. However, he generally found considerable stability of role. The effects of role loss in widowhood were not consistent and were more likely to be the result of other factors surrounding widowhood, such as poverty, ill health and/or very old age, rather than widowhood *per se*. He actually questions the utility of a decremental model of role loss and points instead to a compensation model in which a shifting or realignment of relationships takes place. Older women lose the role of wife but they compensate for this loss by adopting or adapting to other roles. Interestingly, he does not draw on experience across the life-course in this discussion but focuses on current rather than past roles. Anne Martin-Matthews (1991: 9) questions the usefulness of role theory and uses instead a symbolic interactionist approach in order to be: 'Better able to ascertain the basis of responses to bereavement and widowhood and to account for factors that role theory cannot adequately consider.' By using this approach, she looks at the redefinition of the attitudes of others as well as the older woman herself that brings about change in later life widowhood. She starts to explore widowhood from the point of view of older women themselves and the society in which they live. This has the advantage of acknowledging diversity and recognising the structured nature of widowhood.

A body of literature exists which sees widowhood as a major stressful life event (see Holmes and Rahe, 1967). Anne Martin-Matthews (1991) informs us that a major characteristic of Canadian widowhood research is its stress-related nature, with a focus on the *event* of becoming a widow. More recently, Nieboer *et al.* (1995) refer to the loss of a spouse as the life event which requires most adjustment. British research reflects a similar picture (Marris, 1958; Torrie, 1975; Bowling and Cartwright, 1982). The difficulty with this approach is that it focuses on a particular point in time in which the 'event' occurs rather than on the older woman herself and the continuities and discontinuities she brings to that event. Consequently, the event and thus the older widow become pathologised. Eileen Jones-Porter (1994) suggests that when it is assumed that the death of a spouse is a stressful event researchers are more likely to frame data collection in terms of grieving and coping.

Another body of research focuses on widowhood as a psychosocial transition in which widowhood is seen as a disruption to an accustomed way of life. Individuals will cope differently depending on personality and culture (Kimmel, 1990) and on education and social status (Lopata, 1973). More recently, Susan Pickard's (1994) research in South Wales has suggested that this transition can only be understood in the social and geographical context in which it occurs. Fry and Gavrin (1987), in a study of older widows in a homogeneous stable community, also stressed the context of community for defining the experience of widowhood. Here again, the focus is on discontinuity, but I would suggest that the disruption under discussion is bereavement rather than the ongoing or long-term nature of widowhood.

Increasingly, research on older widows is beginning to consider issues of reciprocity and/or exchange. In this model, older women are not seen as powerless victims. Social exchange theory (Toni Antonucci, 1985) identifies loss of reciprocity as a condition under which social support may have negative consequences. For example, the support given to older widows, particularly by family, often leaves them in the role of passive recipients, or patients receiving treatment, and can leave them feeling powerless and dependent. Watanabe Greene and Field (1989), who looked at the well-being of older widows linked to support, also found that too much support and lack of reciprocity had a negative effect on the women, perhaps because they felt they had less control. Phyllis Silverman's (1987) work on self-help groups of widows and widowers highlights the importance of mutual exchange and understanding in the development of a new stage of life. In these self-help groups, older widows and widowers provided mutual support and practical help on the basis of reciprocity. Nicholas Babchuk and Trudy Anderson's (1989) comparison of married and widowed women stressed the importance of friendship ties for widows. Dorothy Jerrome's exploration (1981, 1990, 1991) of older women and friendship reminds us that friendship is offered voluntarily on the basis of reciprocity, both in the past and in the present, and thus confers high morale. This focus on reciprocity allows us to see older widows as active participants in their social world and thus builds in the possibility of growth.

Gail Sheehy (1997: 354) draws on the concept of status passage and identifies widowhood as a major 'transformative event' for women of the 'reconstruction generation' in America. Early socialisation had taught these women that they were not complete without a man and had therefore left them unprepared for widowhood. She suggests that the women who undertake this passage successfully see themselves as survivors. While they may experience fear and loneliness at times, they also gain autonomy and a gathering sense of self. She goes on to say: 'These survivors expect to be even more self-confident as they proceed through their sixties, and most look forward to being serene and ready for new challenges' (Sheehy 1997: 355). The women survivors that she interviewed stressed the importance of taking risks and challenging the expectations of others, thereby confronting the mythology and stereotypes of widowhood.

As I indicated in the Introduction, widowhood in later life is an expectation for most older women. As such, it is an 'on-time' experience. Bernice Neugarten and her colleagues (Neugarten *et al.*, 1965; Neugarten and Datan, 1973; Neugarten, 1977) have explored the existence of a social clock, a system of age norms, that is superimposed on the biological clock. She suggests that we use this 'social clock' to assess ourselves in relation to others and to ask 'How am I doing for my age?' and 'How am I doing compared with others of my cohort?'. This may not make the actual 'event' of widowhood any easier for older women, particularly during the period of bereavement, but it may ultimately have an impact on their understanding of the experience and the possibilities offered. Clearly, there will be generational differences between 'young, old' and 'old, old' women and there may well be different expectations of different life stages (see Chapter

1). Contrary to popular mythology, it may also mean that many older couples will have discussed the probability of one of them dying and may even have made arrangements. Gerontological literature reminds us that in general older people are much more likely to talk about the prospect of dying than their younger counterparts (see, for example, Lieberman and Tobin, 1983).

Widowhood therefore is an ongoing process which happens to a particular individual and takes place within the context of a particular family and a particular community. It has a history that will affect the subsequent life of the older woman. In addition, we cannot ignore the fact that all of this takes place within a societal and political context, which will affect both the objective and subjective experience of widowhood. Older widows have stories to tell about their lives and we must be prepared to hear their voices. Eileen Jones-Porter (1994: 33) suggests that we need a fresh perspective on the life world of older widows, one that is sensitive to the totality of older women's lives and is 'grounded in conversation with older widows'.

An alternative approach

The literature on later life widowhood tells us very little about the *actual experience* of being a widow in late twentieth century Britain. I would suggest this is because of the theoretical perspectives used and confusion of ongoing widowhood with the acute state of bereavement. Experience is not static; it is in the present but it is also in the past. It is something that happens but it is also the process of something happening. It describes the feelings that the individual has as a result of the process, and what has happened. It is, therefore, past and present coming together. Clearly, the use of a biographical approach is significant if these many aspects of experience are to be explored. Experience is also both subjective and objective in that the individual experience is structured by the society in which we live. Widowhood and widowerhood in later life are very different experiences – for example, older men who are widowed tend to remarry fairly quickly after the death of their spouse or they die (Sheehy, 1997), whereas older widows are much more likely to live alone for many years. Older women also suffer the double jeopardy of ageism and sexism (Miriam Bernard and Kathy Meade, 1993a). Dorothy Jerrome (1993) reminds us that for a woman the loss of a partner through death involves a series of losses, which include companionship, material support, a partner in a world which is couple orientated and someone to negotiate on the woman's behalf in a male-dominated society.

The links between feminism and gerontology offer us some possibilities as a way forward. The acknowledgement of the gendered nature of later life is fairly recent in gerontology; what might be tentatively termed a 'feminist gerontology' has begun to emerge (see Shulamit Reinharz, 1986; Arber and Ginn, 1991; Bernard and Meade, 1993a; Diane Gibson, 1996) and is one of the recurring themes in this book. Shulamit Reinharz (1992) suggests that underlying all feminist research is the tenet that all women's lives are important. She says:

> For feminist researchers, females are worth examining as individuals and people whose experience is interwoven with other women. In other words, feminists are interested in women as individuals and as a social category.
>
> (Reinharz, 1992: 24)

Feminist gerontology is now recognising this in relation to older women. We are beginning to explore and understand the impact of gender in later life, at both an individual and societal level. Diane Gibson (1996) tells us that the study of older women, and by implication older widows, has been defined by a preoccupation with male and mid-life perspectives and a tendency to see older women in terms of problems. She says:

> It is my contention that the particular lens through which older women have come to be viewed is one that selectively includes only certain aspects of being old and female.
>
> (Gibson, 1996: 94)

We need to move away from a theoretical perspective such as 'role loss', which defines older women in relation to men. A feminist perspective on later life widowhood offers the possibility of understanding the social reality of later life widowhood via the actresses involved. If we are to truly understand the experience of later life widowhood, we need to transform prevailing gerontological knowledge paradigms to incorporate these older women's lives. Kathryn Anderson *et al.* (1987: 119) in their discussion of feminist methodology in oral history stress the importance of finding out about women's *actual* lives, which: 'Deepens the critique of existing knowledge by documenting the inadequacy of past assumptions.'

A biographical approach to later life widowhood allows us to find out about women's lives from their own perspective. Most of the women in my research have spoken of their need to re-evaluate their lives now that they are widows. Johnson (1978) reminds us of the uniqueness of the human biography. The process of giving a life history is not simply someone telling their story. It is a particular interaction between two people which will vary with different interviewers at different times. By talking about the past and the present, they are enabled to make sense of their current situation; as the researcher, I have had the privilege of gaining an insight into the experience of later life widowhood by listening to their stories. Life histories bring out not only the process of life but also each individual's perspective on their life (Sylvana Di Gregorio, 1986). The starting point in this type of research is the older woman herself – in my own study, it was the twenty women who participated in the research. A life history approach acknowledges the importance of older women's experiences throughout their lives and, as Joanna Bornat (1993) suggests, reveals the differences that older women bring to later life. Earlier experiences may account for ways in which major life changes, such as widowhood, are managed.

The diverse experience of later life widowhood

By drawing on my own empirical research, I propose to discuss the experience of later life widowhood as explored with me by the twenty women who participated in the research. Although they speak as individuals and not as 'group representatives', they nonetheless describe themselves as widows and identify with other widows. In this way, their stories provide us with an insight into the lived experience of a group of older women whose lives are normally hidden away. Consent has been gained from all the participants concerning the names used in this chapter.

The women were all interviewed in their own homes at a time to suit them. Transcriptions of the interview were given back to each of them and an opportunity was provided to make changes and reflect on what had been said. The majority of the women welcomed this opportunity for a further discussion and expressed considerable satisfaction at taking part in the study (see Chambers, 1998). For all of them, it was the first time they had talked openly about their life history and their experiences in widowhood; by telling their story to an eager listener, they were able to make sense of scattered events. Valerie Yow (1994: 17) suggests that this validation is particularly important to people, such as older women, who are devalued by society. In discussing the transcription with Joan, she felt able to say: 'Well, it made me feel stronger because I thought, well I did do that.'

Sylvia also felt validated by telling and subsequently reading her story:

> …I quite enjoyed it, it helped me; it seemed to relieve me, I've never talked to anybody like this before, well you don't… And I thought, well I've always got that [the transcription] now, when I'm on my own I can sit and read it…things came back that I thought I'd put to the back of my mind, I was able to put in place..

So what do these women tell us about their subjective experience of later life widowhood and how does this experience compare with the popular mythology? By using primarily the voices of a selection of the women who participated in the research, I propose to explore each of the myths in turn.

Older widows are a homogeneous group

The women who have participated in my research were all widowed after the age of 55 (the age at which widowhood becomes an 'on-time' experience) and have been widowed for more than 5 years (do not identify themselves as being in bereavement). The sample was voluntary and purposive and, although not representative, provides us with a snapshot of the heterogeneity of later life widowhood in the area in which they lived. Some of the women were known to me previously, others were contacted via a second party, others contacted me because they had heard about the research and wished to participate.

All the women were residing in a variety of settings in Stockport; these included a residential home, sheltered accommodation, purpose-built retirement homes, local authority housing, housing association flats and private housing. Their financial circumstances varied considerably both now and in the past. Several of the women talked about the need to be 'careful' with money since their only source of income was a state pension (and for some income support); others described themselves as 'financially secure', having been 'well provided for' by their husbands. Their educational levels covered a wide spectrum, ranging from leaving school as soon as possible without any qualifications to undertaking higher education. Several of the women returned to education to undertake part-time courses at different levels. Some of the women had never worked outside the family home, whereas others had juggled domestic work and paid work for most of their lives. One of the women described herself as Asian, another woman described herself as having a long-term disability as a result of childhood polio. Three of the women never had children; one of the three helped to raise her niece and had an ongoing, close relationship with the niece and her family. Three of the women had married men much older than themselves. One of the women was in an established relationship with a new male partner, but had chosen not to remarry. Another woman had begun a new relationship with a male partner, but was uncertain about the future. Three of the women spent a lot of time with siblings who lived nearby. Their ages ranged from 64 years to 89 years, thus spanning a number of cohorts. They did, however, all situate themselves historically as belonging to the 'pre-Second World War' generation. Clearly, even within this small sample, the label 'widow' covers extremely diverse experiences and circumstances.

Widowhood is synonymous with the acute state of bereavement

None of the women chose to be widows and most of them vividly remembered their feelings during bereavement. It was a time of sadness, bewilderment, feelings of hopelessness and often loss of confidence:

> My life completely changed…until you are widowed you can't imagine what it's like; it is completely different than I thought it would be…it sapped my confidence.
>
> (Vera)

Betty vividly described her feelings at the time:

> You feel as though…well it's very strange really, it's as though half has been chopped off you, yes, and it's all raw down one side, that's the feeling I got.

However, they were all very aware of the difference between that time and their lives now. They were all able to recall the period of bereavement and talk about the changes that have occurred since that time:

> It doesn't continue [that feeling], it passes eventually. You don't forget but the edges get rubbed off. I suppose after twelve months and by three years most women have got over the worst.
>
> (Betty)

> At first I just wanted to stay in black and be a widow and then I thought, no you've got to pull yourself together. Everything was in a cocoon and you had to come out of it…yes, yes, I suddenly thought I must slip out of this cocoon quick…I started setting the table…I made myself have a main meal at the table once a week…
>
> (Ellen)

And now:

> …it's opened up a great freedom for me…it's very important; I mean I've never had freedom. I mean from joining the army, from being in school and then joining the army at 17 and a half, you were under the control of people, then you got married and you're under control, then you have children and you're under control, and so forth, right the way through. And so I've never really had freedom. It's the first freedom I've ever really had and that's why I think I enjoy it.
>
> (Ellen)

For Farzana, there were differences between the period of bereavement and now. At first, because she still had the responsibility of two unmarried children, she felt overwhelmed. However, it got easier:

> Well at first it all seems very different when you are a widow but then you get used to the life of being a widow and handling all the responsibility.

Elizabeth talked about the role of others during bereavement:

> At first everybody, for a while makes an effort to get you to join in and then gradually you are on your own...I don't think it worried me unduly. If I felt I wanted to go out I'd take myself into...[the town] or something on the train...I can do things on my own.

Eunice stressed the importance of on-time as opposed to off-time experiences. Her daughter had died in her early twenties, a number of years before her husband:

> I think I really went through my worst time when I lost my daughter. You can accept the fact that you lose a husband, he was sixty one. But when I lost my daughter, I found that very difficult.

She felt that her previous bereavement had also prepared her in some ways for her husband's death; in practical terms she was prepared and she knew she would survive the experience.

Widowhood is an experience isolated from the rest of women's lives

All of the women talked about the importance of past experiences and how these had had an impact on their current lives. Widowhood was another chapter in their lives, but certainly not separate from what had gone before. Eunice worked for a voluntary organisation, participated in church activities and had been active in the community for a significant part of her married life. She continued to be active within these organisations. These roles gave her autonomy in her marriage and provided continuity in widowhood.

Ellen joined the Auxiliary Territorial Service (ATS) at 17 and felt that it was a significant part of her life in the past and contributed to her current experience. She met her husband in the army and maintained very strong links with her local organisation, where she has many friends. She said: 'It was a wonderful experience, I think we all got a lot out of the forces...I often say we grew up in a few weeks.' She felt that she learnt to be independent in the ATS and that this served her well in widowhood. The ATS was still a major part of her life:

> When Christmas comes I think I must get about two hundred and fifty cards. We go to [the town] Legion for our meeting and if we finish our meeting we say it's too early to go home yet so go for a cup of tea somewhere…and there's usually about twenty of us…there's a great friendship between the association.

Elizabeth left home at the age of 16 to be a kitchen maid and from an early age saw life as an adventure. She resisted pressure to marry until she felt she was ready to do so. During the war years, her husband was away from her and her young daughter for 4 years. She talked about when he came back:

> Well it was wonderful really but there was one thing, you had been in control all those years…it took some adjusting. You get to rely on yourself and you cope…I've always been independent I think…

This independence and positive approach to life continued in widowhood. Despite increasing disability, she regularly undertook long train journeys to visit friends and family and enjoyed the freedom of living alone.

Patricia's husband worked nights for 35 years of their married life. This and the fact that he was 16 years older than her clearly had, and continued to have, an impact on her daily life. She had never had a close friend – any friends they had earlier in married life were his friends – and she acknowledged that she did not really know how to make friends. She was lonely in widowhood and very dependent on her daughter. In my conversations with her, it became very apparent that this loneliness and dependence on her daughter had also been a feature of her married life.

Bee had married, in her late twenties, a man who was much older than herself. She gave up her career on marriage:

> I was determined my marriage was going to be a success…I'd seen what my mother and father had had to struggle through in the 1930s and I was determined my life would not be the same.

She worked hard in her marriage and was financially secure throughout her married life (and continued to be). She was able to build up a strong social life which revolved around her passions for golf and bridge. She and her husband had discussed the possibility of his death and had made sure she knew all there was to know about the house and their finances. She remained in the house that she had lived in all her married life and had maintained strong ties with friends, neighbours and the golf club:

> I knew everything I had to do in the house because he had said to me this is something you've got to know, to look after...so I just got on with it...I had my golf and my bridge and my friends.

Jenny was very aware of both continuities and discontinuities in widowhood and that the experience is not static. Talking about her best friend, she said:

> Although she was a friend before John died...it's different now. We are much closer now. I didn't have a best friend while I was married, John was my best friend. You don't have a best friend when you are married. Our friendship is much deeper now.

She felt that many of the skills she acquired earlier on in life had served her well:

> I was always the organiser, I always sorted the bills out. I do a lot more now [for myself]...I had to do quite a lot for John before he died. I had to help him bath and wash... My life would have been very different if John were alive.

Older widows are not self-determining

Many of the women talked about widowhood offering them an opportunity to determine the course of their lives more than they had been able to in the past. They felt that they had become more proactive and less reactive.

For Edith, the death of her husband was an extremely traumatic experience, following on from the death of her mother and then her brother. She felt bereft and alone and she suffered from clinical depression, which resulted in her admission to hospital. However, 5 years on, she felt that she had gained control of her life and was able to make choices about her future. She lived in a retirement flat that she bought 3 years after her husband died. She said:

> I did it all on my own...I'd never done anything like it before...I mean I didn't have to do anything. I didn't have to pay a bill. Donald did all of that sort of thing...I had all the bedrooms fitted. I had to get rid of all my furniture and buy all new furniture, apart from the unit and the rug that Donald had bought. Now I can buy things that are to my taste...I

do think I have more confidence now than before. I look forward to the future.

Doris also talked about an increase in self-determination. She acknowledged that her husband had been a very domineering man throughout their married life. She said:

> He [her husband] was very stubborn. If he didn't want to do something he wouldn't, so as soon as he died I felt I could please myself now. It was the first time in my life that I could please myself.

She had made choices about where she lived and how she spent her money: 'For the first time in my life I'm doing what I want and it's so nice…it is liberating, it really is. And at my age as well.' She was aware that her life would have been very different had her husband survived his illness as she would have been his principal carer: 'I was relieved that my husband went as quickly as he did. He would have been a terrible patient.'

Feelings are also part of the experience of being in charge of one's life, and all the women expressed their feelings about widowhood. Jenny commented that:

> I'm not often lonely. Sometimes when I'm not feeling well but I snap out of it. I can always phone my friend. I keep busy. I think the activity helps and being healthy.

Ellen, too, talked about her busy social life:

> I don't make my life a misery. In fact I quite enjoy my life. I always think, well he would have enjoyed his life. We always said whichever one went first the other wasn't to mope, you've got to get on with your life.

However, a number of the women perceived the vulnerability of being an older woman alone:

> When Stan died I used to leave a little light on in the kitchen…one on in the living room…one on at the top of the stairs which I'd never done before in my life…that was how I felt.
>
> (Katherine)

Eunice identified the stigma attached to the label 'widow' and felt that, initially, she experienced problems being in control of her own life. She felt that she was at the mercy of others ready to exploit her supposed vulnerability:

> One thing I hated first of all when I first lost my husband was the word 'widow'…I had to have a new garage door and a salesman came along and when he discovered I was a widow, this label you know, I think he felt I was easy picking. Women on their own are very vulnerable.

As her confidence increased, she felt less vulnerable and no longer stigmatised by the label: 'I don't think the label bothers me as much now.' She felt that she was in control of her life and was able to make choices and decisions which determined her future.

Older widows are lonely and isolated

All of the women were enmeshed in relationships with family and friends. These relationships were all different, depending on their personal circumstances and life histories. They acknowledged that often they were alone (most of them lived alone) and sometimes they were lonely, but only two of them described their lives as lonely and isolated. These two women both felt that loneliness and isolation had been features of their married lives and had more to do with their life history than their current status.

Most of the women recognised that there had been changes from their married lives, particularly concerning the development of friendships with other widowed or ever-single women and their relationships with 'couple' friends.

Concerning other 'single' women, Ellen said:

> I think you do sort of cling to one another, people who are on their own rather than go to a couple. I don't think it's the married people, I think it's the people who are single, they do think they are getting in the way.

During a busy working life, nursing and then running a Blackpool boarding house, Evelyn had little time for friendships outside her marriage. In widowhood, she was able develop a close friendship with a woman whom previously she had only known as a neighbour:

> Jenny was the best friend I've had in my adult life. Although we were neighbours we didn't get to know each other until our husbands died. We used to go out together before but not as real friends. We always knew the other was there when we needed someone. At that time, it was more important than my family.

Most of the women acknowledged changes in their relationships with married friends. The year after her husband died, Eunice went on a Saga holiday on her own. She met a lot of other widows there who warned her that her married friends would gradually disappear. She found that this only partially proved to be the case, some friendships had continued, others had ended.

For Edith, the death of her husband was made worse by the loss of 'couple' friends: 'When my husband was alive it was all Donald and Edith this and that, but it's amazing when he died they didn't want to know me.' However, this had been compensated for by the development of new friendships and new activities. She said about these new friendships:

> …that is really important, people accepting me as Edith. It's a big thing. You don't forget some of your old friends and I don't mean to forget Donald, but now all the friends I've made and believe me I've made lots of new friends, they accept me as Edith.

For Bee, the experience had been entirely different:

> When you are left on your own and you've had a good social life, you feel a bit lost and don't know what to do. And it's things like holidays, you think how am I going to cope. But the nice thing was they all said, come with us Bee…and they were all married couples…most of my friends are couples.

In a couple-orientated society, older widows are often perceived as lonely because they are without a partner. Further, it is often assumed that the reason many older widows do not remarry is because of the lack of available older men. There were a variety of relationships and attitudes to remarriage among the women in the study.

Sylvia had a new partner, 9 years older than herself, whom she had met fairly soon after the death of her husband. She felt that this relationship was very different from her marriage: 'I really am very happy again. I love him very much. But it's a different type of love than I had for James.' She did acknowledge the possibility that her partner may die before her and wondered how she would cope, but had decided that she would take the risk: 'You can't go through life thinking like that.'

Eunice acknowledged that she missed the company of men, but had no wish to remarry:

> I've missed male company…some people approach dating agencies but I've never done that. If I had met somebody I would have enjoyed

their company but I don't think I'd have married them…I do miss male companionship.

A number of years after the death of her husband, Joan met another man, who subsequently died. She felt that during the time that she was with him there were opportunities to socialise which were not available to a woman on her own. She described widowhood as: 'A tremendous loss socially, because we'd loved ballroom dancing and suddenly I'd no one to go with. Oh you do feel very different.' However, during that relationship, they maintained separate homes and spent time apart, pursuing different activities with separate friends.

Many of the women expressed the view that they did not wish to remarry. There was a feeling among some that they did not wish to go through another bereavement or that they could not replace their partner, but for others, such as Jenny, there was a strong feeling of positive choice about staying single:

> I've had an offer, a professor from the university. We'd both been married the same length of time and been widowed. But I didn't want to. Marriage ties you down, I wouldn't want that. If you marry someone it's because you want to be together. He's married now and I'm friends with him and his new wife. Ada asks me if I feel I've missed my chance…but I don't feel I have. It's not what I want.

Widowhood is a period of decline

Many of the women expressed satisfaction with their quality of life and challenged the view that widowhood is a period of decline. They acknowledged that many changes had occurred in their lives.

Eunice reflected on life in widowhood:

> I definitely think I have grown…I think you get things in perspective, you sort out what's important and you realise life is never the same but you are strengthened…there is a certain freedom and it's no disrespect to your partner to feel that.

Jenny talks about her very active social life:

> I go out a lot…I've a friend Ada we go on holiday together…we've had some lovely holidays. I've even been paragliding…after John died I used to go to swimming lessons and learned to swim…they put this harness on me and I went up in the air…I spend a lot of time doing

things with the church, I visit people, I play scrabble with Gladys at [a local elderly persons' home] every Saturday. I go out with friends for meals, for our birthdays.

In widowhood, Jean resumed dancing, something she had loved when she was younger but had 'temporarily' given up during her married life:

I danced until I got married and then I had the children and went out to work, there's no time for dancing then. I didn't do any until I came here to the club.

With her friend, another widow, Jean was instrumental in setting up the dancing class at her local over-sixties club. Her excitement and enjoyment of life was apparent when she talked about dancing and the club.

Despite her very difficult period of bereavement, Edith felt that in widowhood she was more confident and assertive. Reiterating the point she made earlier, she said:

I do think I have more confidence and I can do more than before…Like my car insurance came this morning and I nearly died at the price of it. Well, before I would have accepted that but now I can say, you've got to find me another quote.

Whereas previously her husband had always organised the family holiday, it was Edith who now organised holidays and weekends away for friends and neighbours and took great delight in this new role.

A number of the women were aware of differences between their own experiences and those of 'still married' friends, and some of them felt that they had more freedom to take up opportunities than their married counterparts. Jenny remarked that: 'I have friends who are married and we do things together but often she won't because of her husband.' Betty, too, talking about her friendship with a woman in her drama group who had been recently widowed, contrasted life as a married woman with life as a single woman:

Well, we've always been good friends but of course she was married and her husband was a bit demanding because he wasn't well for many years and we didn't realise it and she was always saying, 'I must go Ted will be wondering where I am.' Whereas now, I feel she is making choices and asserting herself where she couldn't before…I wonder how many women find that when they are widows?

Challenging the stereotype

What begins to emerge when we listen to older widows talking about their present lives is, first, the difference that older women bring to later life and, second, how their experience is shaped both by their own life experiences and the expectations of others. For all of the women, there were many continuities and fewer discontinuities. The continuities included family ties, friendship, residence, social interests, multiplicity of roles, financial issues as well as loneliness and lack of confidence for some women.

The discontinuities included poor health, solo living, vulnerability and loss of friends. Yet, it is often the discontinuities which are highlighted in the mythology surrounding widowhood. Diane Gibson (1996: 438) suggests that this reinforces the view that older women are a problem; we see their difficulties, but: 'Comparatively little is made, however, of the closer instrumental and affective ties that the [widowed] women experience with family and friends.' All of the women were participating in networks of family and friends and all of them saw themselves as contributing to a greater or smaller extent to those networks. They all felt that after an initial period of bereavement their lives had continued to develop and they had individually continued to grow. On the whole, they saw themselves as active participants rather than passive onlookers.

Their experience of widowhood at the time of interview was clearly affected by their past experience. Patricia, for example, described herself as very lonely and friendless in widowhood, and yet in discussing her life history revealed that she had been lonely for most of her married life. Those women who had been more autonomous earlier on in the life-course, such as Elizabeth and Eunice, and who had a strong sense of self had a different experience from some of their contemporaries who struggled in widowhood to achieve a new sense of 'I'.

What is very clear from the interviews with these women is that their experiences were very diverse but individually they were able to make sense of that experience in their own terms. They were also aware that others, sometimes family or neighbours but rarely friends, may see them as vulnerable and lonely.

Conclusion

Some of the myths surrounding widowhood in later life have been challenged in this chapter by listening to women talking about their lives. The women who participated in the research all had a story to tell and all seemed very aware that they had undergone a transition to another phase in their life, a phase which they had changed. By telling their story, they felt validated and were able to begin to make sense of their lives; they felt able to talk about positive aspects of their lives as well as those areas which caused them distress. Subsequent cohorts of older widows will have experienced very different collective and individual life histories which may well include divorce and remarriage. They will have come of age during a time when women's rights were openly discussed, when marriage and motherhood were not necessarily seen as a lifetime career. How will this impact on their experience of later life widowhood? Future research about such 'silent' groups of older women needs to listen to their voices and enable them to challenge 'taken for granted' assumptions about their lives.

9 Older women, long-term marriage and care

Mo Ray

Introduction

Long-term marriage constitutes a highly important social, emotional, financial and practical relationship. Despite the significance of the relationship, long-term marriage remains an under-researched area, particularly in Britain. Janet Askham (1995) has suggested that the comprehensive study of marriage from the perspective of older people has been neglected, in part, as a result of it being concerned with older people, who are seen as marginal to society's mainstream projects.

The significant contribution made by older women, and men, in the provision of informal care, most particularly provided on a co-resident basis to their spouses, is also often overlooked. Their relative invisibility, in comparison with caregivers in other parts of the life-course, may serve to reinforce the myth that very old women and men are inevitably a burden on the state and their family members. Sara Arber and Jay Ginn (1991) demonstrated, in their reanalysis of the General Household Survey, that older people provide 35% of the total volume of informal care to people aged 65 or over and nearly 50% of co-resident care of older men and women. Based on available evidence, spouse care is likely to remain the most reliable and predictable form of informal care (Janet Finch, 1995). On the face of it, the care-giving literature appears to offer a vast array of published research. But, research which focuses specifically on long-term marriage relationships is much less common than explorations of other familial relationships. There is also an almost complete absence of care-giving research which considers the process of managing the challenges associated with emerging chronic illness from *both* partners' perspectives (Gillian Parker, 1994).

Based on research for my own doctoral study, this chapter discusses the impact of chronic illness on long-term marriage relationships. It is organised into three main sections. First, I assess the contribution of some of the key literature about both long-term marriage and spousal care-giving. Second, I discuss certain aspects of my own research material within the context of a process that I term 'reorganisation'. I consider how participants define and construct new roles and responsibilities which may be associated with 'caring' and I highlight the diverse ways in which participants provided support and how those roles changed, sometimes fundamentally, over time. The chapter concludes with a brief discussion of the research outcomes in relation to published research on long-term marriage and spousal caring relationships.

Myself and my research

My interest in long-term marriage relationships in the context of chronic illness and disability stems from personal and professional experience. As a young adult, my grandfather gave up full-time employment to care for my grandmother, who had multi-infarct dementia. The sorts of issues I pondered were how, or indeed whether, my grandparents' individual and marital identities could be preserved and maintained when relationship norms and routines that were taken for granted become destabilised and unsettled.

My experience as a social worker also suggests that, as a professional group, we are not always good at working with the diversity of biography and the strengths, skills and aspirations that long-married couples use to manage and make sense of the challenges that they face. An increasing focus on managing finite resources through, for example, eligibility criteria may lead to reductionist approaches to assessments of need (Parton, 1996) which are more concerned with procedural matters and less concerned with considering the assessed person in the context of their biography, relationships, strengths and skills.

These two areas formed the basis of my interest. I was interested to see how participants' marriage biographies were used to explain the ways in which they managed their current, often very difficult, circumstances. What use did people make of the continuities they perceived as important in their relationships, and how did they maintain or reconstruct marriage identities in the face of significant change? These research questions formed the basis of my study.

The chapter is based on a qualitative study with thirteen couples married for 35 years or more. I used tape-recorded in-depth interviews first with the couple and afterwards individually. I visited participants again 6 months later for follow-up interviews to gain insight into the way transitions and new challenges had occurred in the intervening time, and into the strategies that couples had used to manage them. I spoke with participants in detail about their marital biographies and present circumstances. Using grounded theory as a method of analysis, I worked on developing conceptual categories which reflected the strategies and approaches that couples use to manage the transitions and challenges associated with chronic illness and disability.

The study upon which this chapter is based focuses upon the experience of long-married *couples*. Although the emphasis in this chapter is on the experiences of married women, it is neither possible nor desirable effectively to separate women's experiences from the men with whom they had enduring lifelong relationships. Instead, the aim of this chapter is to explore the nature of relationships and the ways in which long-established marital norms, usually shaped by traditional expectations about divisions of labour, power and position, were forced into change by the experience of illness.

Examining the literature

To provide the best opportunity for exploring chronic illness in the context of long-term marriage, two bodies of research are examined. They focus on long-term marriage and on spousal care-giving. Of necessity, the literature reviewed in this present chapter is not exhaustive (for comprehensive reviews, see for example Brubaker, 1990; Parker, 1990; Askham *et al.*, 1992; Julia Twigg, 1992; Askham, 1994, 1995; Nolan *et al.*, 1996; Twigg and Atkin, 1994).

Long-term marriage: a limited research agenda?

The research that is available generally suggests that marriage results in positive outcomes in terms of health and well-being (for example Hess and Soldo, 1985), although the relative advantage is reported as greater for men than women. Women may also evaluate their marriage as less happy than their male counterparts. The reason for this is not entirely clear, but some suggestion has been made that women are likely to be more idealistic in their relationship expectations (Atchley, 1992). Exploration of the ways in which power, access to resources and the way in which relationships are structured and organised have hardly been considered in relation to long-term marriage, and so explanations of gendered difference in this direction remain speculative.

The most significant body of research, coming from North America, has focused on evaluating levels of 'marital satisfaction' or understanding what factors contribute to satisfaction. Much of this research was historically conducted within the framework of the family life cycle (Rosalyn Schram, 1979).The basic proposition is that marital satisfaction is influenced by the tasks and responsibilities typically undertaken at various points in the family's development, and research has examined marital satisfaction on the basis of this hypothesis (for example Rollins and Feldman, 1970; Janette Copeland *et al.*, 1984; Herman, 1994).

Despite considerable research attention, the heterogeneous nature of these studies, samples, variables and methods of assessment result in a diverse and inconclusive mix of findings (Sporakowski and Axelson, 1984). One major difficulty with the research is that it is predicated around the notion that there can be a 'global' evaluation of marital satisfaction (Sporakowski and Axelson, 1984). Despite its potential attraction as a 'catch all' term that has been widely used, critics have questioned the utility of the concept of marital satisfaction as a research tool (Johnson *et al.*, 1986). Many of these studies also use cross-sectional research designs, so they are unable to capture change over time adequately. Moreover, the studies invariably use different criteria to operationalise definitions of marital satisfaction, making comparisons problematic. Finally, analysis of results usually refers to married couples, but the data are rarely analysed on the basis of matched couples. While participants may be married, there is no guarantee that they are married to each other.

Long-term marriage and divisions of labour

There is a further significant body of research aimed at examining the patterning of responsibility for various aspects of domestic divisions of labour within long-term marriage. The research available in this area is again inconclusive. Some general, if rather mixed, trends appear to emerge. Some theorists (for example Brubaker, 1985) propose that gendered orientations to divisions of labour in later life are influenced by a reduction in role differentiation between men and women. Lois Tamir and Toni Antonucci (1981) comment that after retirement men appeared to develop more affiliative behaviours and orientations in marriage. Women, on the other hand, tend to become more independent and shift attention away from their spouse and family. Some research has also suggested that men take on more 'feminine' tasks in older age (for example Pat Keith *et al.*, 1981, 1992), whereas other research has concluded that sex role differentiation is maintained throughout older age as a relationship continuity (for example Norah Keating and Priscilla Cole, 1980; Maxine Szinovacz, 1980; Brubaker and Hennon, 1982). Brubaker (1985) concludes that there is a considerable amount of sharing of domestic tasks, but responsibility for them remains within traditional domains of organisation. Other studies have revealed similar overall findings in that couples share some activities, although they generally maintain traditional divisions of labour unless illness or disability forces a change (for example Timothy Brubaker and Linda Ade-Ridder, 1986; Ade-Ridder and Brubaker, 1988; Keith *et al.*, 1992). Jennifer Mason's (1987) qualitative study concluded that a fundamental renegotiation of gendered responsibilities is unlikely to occur in later life. She argued:

> Through the payment of lip service to women's domestic power, the ultimate orchestration of power of husbands, over their wives, stemming from their socially advantaged position, can be concealed whilst also being reinforced.
>
> (Mason, 1987: 102)

Much of the division of labour research, however, does not deal with the potential complexities that inform and influence how divisions of labour are sustained, or under what circumstances they are renegotiated. The research also takes place outside any theoretical framework and makes little comment about how traditionally ascribed divisions of labour reinforce power imbalances between wives and husbands.

More recently, there has been some qualitative research aimed at looking at processes in the marriage relationship, such as communication strategies and the ways in which couples construct marital identities (for example Fran Dickson, 1991; Alford-Cooper, 1998). Dickson (1991), for example, highlights the ways in which communication and interaction reveal different types and levels of emotional closeness and proximity in long-lasting marriages. Alford-Cooper's work (1998) highlights the importance of biography and cohort membership in influencing the ways in which marriage relationships may be defined and constructed at different points in history. However, qualitative exploration of long-term marriage still remains an underinvestigated area.

Spousal care-giving: diverse research trends

Over the past two decades, there has been an enormous proliferation of care-giving research. An underlying theme informing much of this work on care-giving is that caring for an ill person is inherently stressful or burdensome, and considerable research effort has been directed towards understanding the causes and consequences that the experience of care-giving burden has on people providing informal care. A review of the literature reveals how commonplace it has been to associate care-giving with the notion of burden (Schulz, 1990). Researchers have even questioned the utility of publishing further research in this area without reconsidering the theoretical frameworks and empirical approaches which underpin it (for example Zarit, 1989). The emphasis on burden research can have the effect of reinforcing the myth of the inevitability of older people becoming a burden and this is particularly sharply focused on older women, as highlighted in Chapter 3. More recently, research has begun to explore some of the positive aspects of engaging in caring relationships (for example Nolan *et al.*, 1996).

However, the person being cared for and the context of the relationship in which caring occurs remain marginalised in research terms (Parker, 1994).

A review of some of the spousal care-giving research yields a diverse range of findings. There is research evidence to suggest that the nature and extent of care recipients' cognitive and behavioural difficulties are important predictive variables in the experience of burden (for example Amanda Barusch and Wanda Spaid, 1989; Margaret Wallhagen, 1992). Research focusing attention on the nature of the relationship between caregiver and care recipient has also suggested that spouses find their role more stressful when compared with other types of relationship (for example Zarit *et al.*, 1986). This is further influenced by the tendency for spouses providing care to co-reside with their partners and to provide care for longer periods of time. Moreover, the loss of a partner as an important emotional and social support may add to the experience of burden. Other research, however, has reported that spouses providing care experience less burden and conflict when compared with other care-giving relationships (for example Rosalie Young and Eva Kahana, 1989). Research focusing on the emotional consequences of care-giving has highlighted feelings of loss and isolation for the spousal caregiver (for example Phyllis Braudy-Harris, 1993; Parsons, 1997).

A significant and consistent theme is that women carers experience more stress and burden than their male counterparts (for example Miller and Cafasso, 1992). However, reported gender differences are complicated by other research which suggests that, in terms of burden, men and women may actually report similar subjective experiences. Yet other researchers have argued that observed gender differences are confounded by the age variable, i.e. women spouse carers in research samples tend to be younger than their male counterparts and experience the role as inherently burdensome and 'off time' (for example Barusch and Spaid, 1989; Rachael Pruchno and Nancy Resch, 1989). The meta-analysis by Miller and Cafasso (1992) of fourteen descriptive studies found no statistically significant gender differences. They speculate that a social role hypothesis – that caregivers respond to the demands required of them – is one possible explanation.

Clare Ungerson (1987), in her qualitative study of mixed-sex spousal caregivers, generated themes which suggested, for example, that men tended to define motivations for their caring role in terms of love. Women, however, defined their role in terms of duty. Ungerson argues that this differentiation in apparent motives could be an important basis for the explanation of sex differences in the formation of caring relationships. Miller (1987) suggests that men have little difficulty in assuming authority in a care-giving situation, which appears to be perceived as a natural extension of their authority within the family. Women, however, are reported to have considerable difficulty asserting their authority in the care-giving role and, for example, experience problems when their role necessitates telling their husbands what to do.

A number of commentators have critiqued the gender-based literature on care-giving on the basis that it enforces a simplistic dichotomy between women and men (for example Alexis Walker, 1992; Fisher, 1994; Ann Opie, 1994). Walker (1992: 45) comments:

> While it is important to document and describe caring labour, the gender difference approach tends to reify the immutably distinct nature of women and men. Typically, in such an approach, care-giving by women is defined as normative and men's performance is compared to it... This strategy of identifying gender differences understates both the diversity within gender and the similarities between men and women. As recent research has shown, not all sisters approach care-giving in the same way, and some brothers are like some sisters in their care-giving behaviour...

Opie (1994: 37), in a feminist reading of male and female caregivers, challenges the tendency to respond to gender as a 'unified and closed concept' which forces emotional reactions to the care-giving role to be analysed on the basis of sex difference. She maintains that diversity in emotional responses to the care-giving role must be highlighted in order to move research away from simply reaffirming existing gender stereotypes.

Drawing the strands together

My reading of both literatures indicates a consistent overlap in their dominant research methods. Lack of agreement in the way in which key terms such as 'burden' or 'marital satisfaction' have been operationalised may account for the apparently contradictory findings that have been briefly reviewed here. One difficulty in evaluating studies in both areas relates to a tendency to describe findings, rather than to locate the research within theoretical frameworks. Calls have been made in relation to both marriage (for example Brubaker, 1990; Askham, 1995) and care-giving (Parker, 1994; Gubrium, 1995) to provide a sharper focus in relation to the theoretical foundations upon which the research has been built.

It is still the case that relatively little is known about spousal care-giving in the context of marriage and even less in terms of managing disability within long-established marital relationships considering both partners' perspectives (Parker, 1994). Clare Wenger (1990) has identified that the needs of older caregivers, in the context of their relationships, remains a neglected issue. This seems paradoxical given the demonstrated importance of older spouse carers as a 'first line of defence' for their partners experiencing illness or disability (Elenor Palo-Stoller, 1992). In terms of care-giving in the context of married relationships, with significant exceptions (for example Juliet Corbin and Anselm Strauss, 1988; Parker, 1993), there is an absence of studies that examine caring relationships from both partners' perspectives, and in the context of their long-term marriage relationships.

Moreover, the current emphasis on care-giving from just one person's perspective renders the partner with disabilities invisible and essentially passive. This may serve to reinforce stereotyped myths about the experience of disability in later life together with notions about the inevitability of dependency in older age, which has particular relevance to the lives of older women. The emphasis on the burdens of care-giving may also serve to pathologise a partner who provides support (Twigg and Atkin, 1994). A failure to develop holistic and multiple perspectives on the ways that care-giving may be defined and experienced will render the knowledge base narrow in its conception and understanding of the complexities of the role. Focusing on an analysis which searches for a simple dichotomy between female and male difference in caring may overlook the gender equality that appears in caring in later life (Arber and Ginn, 1991) and reify a 'right' way to provide care. Women who do not match up to the picture that much research paints of them as carers may also be in danger of being overlooked.

The study

In my study, I interviewed thirteen couples jointly and individually and then followed these up with joint interviews 6 months after first contact. The rationale for longitudinal follow-up interviews was to try to track the way that new transitions were responded to and managed by participants. As stated earlier, I used grounded theory as a method of research and analysis. My analysis and subsequent write-up covers a range of conceptual categories which focus on the ways in which couples manage the changes and transitions associated with chronic illness and disability. In this chapter, I focus on the development of roles or activities that may be construed as caring. These are fundamentally linked to a process that I call here 'reorganisation'.

Reorganisation refers to the active attempts that couples make to manage disruptions in their established routines, roles or activities caused by the impact of illness or disability. Managing the transition can mean that one partner is often involved in assuming responsibility for new and additional roles which have either been removed from, or relinquished by, the partner experiencing ill health. Alternatively, the reorganisation may involve a spouse providing specific support or assistance to enable their partner to maintain part or all of a role or activity. In this way, long-standing roles or tasks become amended or adapted. The immediate aim of reorganisation strategies is for couples to be able to stabilise a situation which has been destabilised by unpredictable or unanticipated events, circumstances or changes. The ultimate goal is for reorganisation attempts to become stable and assimilated into the domestic organisation as a successful outcome to managing the transition. It is the loss, taking on, adoption or management of tasks or roles that influence, and ultimately shape, the meanings that spouses attribute to this process. Moreover, it is the process of successive reorganisation strategies, over wide-ranging areas of domestic and marital organisation, which creates dynamic and changing caring roles and relationships.

Caring defined

A number of commentators have identified the difficulties associated with defining what constitutes caring (for example Gillian Parker and Dot Lawton, 1990; Arber and Ginn, 1991). Conversely, much of the literature exploring the effects of stress and burden caused by care-giving assumes an unproblematic definition. That is, it appears to be assumed that we know what is meant by care-giving, and this implies a degree of homogeneity which does not, in reality, exist.

In my own study, wives providing additional support and care constructed and defined their roles differently, confirming considerable diversity. For example, a wife may define herself as providing additional roles and tasks commonly associated with caring but continue to emphasise her marriage as the primary relationship. Comments such as, 'he's still my husband' or 'sustaining our marriage is vitally important' highlight the primacy of the relationship. Among my sample, there were two marriage relationships which were significantly affected by ambivalence and marital difficulty. These women stressed the imposition of the duties involved in managing disability against a backdrop of sparse and rapidly declining relationship benefits or unequal exchange (Parker, 1993). Mrs Hockney both spoke of herself as 'a carer' and spontaneously defined her changing relationship as having similarities with mothering (Ungerson, 1987). I pursued this through further interviews with other women participants. Mrs Blake agreed with this way of defining what she did, whereas other women actively disagreed. For both Mrs Hockney and Mrs Blake, identifying similarities with their current role to that of mothering was accentuated in their narratives by the loss of experiences which resonated with their identity as a wife. Instead, both women emphasised the drudgery of domestic work, and the physical care and tending, against minimal reciprocity. In their narratives, their role focused on being 'bossy' with their husbands and taking care of their partners as if they were children. Two extracts from both women's narratives illustrate these points:

M: How would you say you felt in yourself? [about providing support to Harold]

Mrs Hockney: Well I suppose I feel much the same but I feel more like his mother than…in a way mostly, because I've got to boss him about you know 'stand up straight, lock your knees' you know 'don't let your head go down'. This is when I get him out of bed onto the commode for instance. I think that's what's really happened is I've taken over. He's normal really I don't know how to describe it, it's funny, I've taken over more being his mother.

M: Some people say, I mean I've come across people who might say, I'm more like a mother or…a paid nurse or…

Mrs Blake: Oh yes, there's that element very much so. They go from being a grown man to a child. I sometimes think he thinks I'm his mother because I have to tuck him in and what have you and he expects it. He says, 'I haven't had this yet' [in a plaintive voice] or something that you think 'Well, he relies on me for everything, very childlike, he's going back to his childhood'… Yes. He does think I'm his mother at times.

Mrs Clarke agreed that the sorts of tasks she may do for her husband bore similarities to those associated with mothering. She also commented on the way that formal care services treated her husband in a childlike or infantilised way. However, she rejected the notion that she *felt* like a mother to her husband. Mrs Jenkins also rejected the mothering 'label' as an appropriate way to define how she experienced her role. Unlike the other women, she had supported her husband for over a decade and defined her role as a carer who was also a 'devoted wife'. When I asked her, for example, about her *husband's* strengths she said 'he's a very good patient'. Similarly, Mrs Saunders rejected a mothering metaphor, but spent a significant amount of time in her narrative highlighting the many ways in which she brought to the forefront important relationship continuities in the context of living with a very ill partner. This seemed to be a very important aspect of maintaining a marital identity, grounded in continuities which had, in reality, become fragmented by her husband's cognitive impairment.

In some cases, caring was defined as mutual support. Mr and Mrs Day and Mr and Mrs Lynch, for example, focused on the importance of mutual support in managing their circumstances. Neither spouse identified the other as 'a carer': they took care of each other. I, as an outsider, might identify one of them as objectively providing more support than the other, but that is not how they constructed their accounts.

The way caring was defined by the spouses undertaking it was fundamentally linked to perceptions about the nature of the marriage relationship. This was, in turn, linked to the nature of the challenges that managing disability engendered and the potential responses to them.

The diverse range of caring activities

In the context of further defining the nature of caring relationships, an examination of the actual tasks and roles reveals considerable diversity between participants and, when compared across time, with the same participants. In line with much published research, domestic divisions of labour in this study were identified by wives and husbands as being virtually static across married and retirement years. In essence, divisions of labour followed traditional patterns, with wives maintaining and serving the domestic sphere while their partners were wage earners. However, during the research phase, roles and tasks changed to meet the demands that illness and disability engendered. Moreover, once roles and tasks had begun to be influenced by the impact of illness and disability, they often changed considerably across very short time spans.

As I have already highlighted, some couples defined their circumstances, at the time of my contact with them, as taking care of each other. Roles and responsibilities may remain substantially unchanged and couples identified their organisation as mutually supportive. Mr and Mrs Day and Mr and Mrs Lynch illustrated this. For both couples, no clear definition or perception of one person needing to 'do' more to support the other emerged at the first point of contact. Help from outside agencies was arranged for tasks or activities that could not be completed between them. Mr and Mrs Day illustrate an aspect of mutual support:

Mr Day: Well it's a great thing because we rely on each other.
Mrs Day: Well we understand you know what it is to be poorly.
Mr Day: We don't hesitate…I mean to say she'll say to me I'll get you a cup of tea Bob and I say all right Win…four times she might say that to me…it's her brain you see, old age. And in the finish I get up and make it for her and she'll say 'Oh thank you I was just going to get you a cup of tea.' [laughs] That's how it goes on between us see?

A number of participants did not undertake significant levels of the physical or personal tending work most often associated with caring. Mrs Saunders, for example, had mobility difficulties as a result of severe arthritis. Her husband had daily physical and personal care needs which were met by home care services and respite care. Mrs Saunders defined and constructed her role as having significant additional care responsibilities. She identified the primary focus of her role as the provision of social support and stimulation (informed by the importance of biographical knowledge and maintenance of her husband's identity), cooking for her husband and assisting him to eat and monitoring the formal care that he received. The importance she placed on biographical knowledge, emotional support and acting as advocate are illustrated in the following extracts:

> He needs stimulating and people talking to him and things to do which he doesn't get when he's in respite. One of the things I've found he enjoys is paper and letters and notepad and pens. He sits all day long back in his office sorting things and his mind's ticking over, he's moving all day long, his hands are moving, his brain is moving.
> ... So I've made an appointment with the hospital manager at... put her in the picture a bit and she said she agreed I had a problem but when she came back last night, there's nothing... that's it. But they're trying to find some way around the laundry problem and the manager said she'd made sure there was somebody to talk to him but it doesn't work like that because he talks to himself and people get a bit pensive...
> (Mrs Saunders)

The notion of a supportive spouse as someone who evaluates and monitors the care their partner receives was an important element in some participants' definitions of a caring relationship (for example Twigg and Atkin 1994). This role is not surprising for a number of reasons. First, if spouses are themselves unable to undertake new tasks as part of a reorganisation strategy then it is likely that they will be concerned that whoever is going to undertake the new roles does so in an appropriate way. Second, the care and concern for their partners that may have been fostered over a lifetime of marriage is likely to continue as a defining part of their relationship, especially when others are recruited to assist with reorganisation strategies. Finally, based on biographical familiarity and their own ideas about care and standards, the supportive partner is likely to identify themselves as the most appropriate person to monitor the care that their spouse is receiving from an outside agency.

There were also participants in my sample who reported providing significant levels of physical care, supervision and night-time care, together with other practical and emotional support. Mrs Blake, for example, was providing care of this nature for her husband. In her own experience, the changes in her roles and responsibilities caused by her partner's disabilities had built up over a period of time and reflected the dynamic nature of the caring role. She had begun with what she called 'keeping an eye', but this had changed over the course of 2 years as her husband's ability to undertake daily activities independently had altered.

Caring relationships

A common thread running through the narratives of wives was a feeling of responsibility for the well-being of their ill partners. Women too, who were chronically ill, demonstrated an ongoing concern about the well-being of their husbands who provided them with support. The identification of this responsibility occurred regardless of how marriage relationships were evaluated, although this did not inevitably mean that wives felt that they had to be responsible for directly providing all aspects of care and support. Nor did wives receiving care and support expect, or want, it to come entirely from their husbands.

Nevertheless, there was a strong sense from participants that the relationship had been a continuity for good or ill throughout the life-course. As such, there was almost a moral imperative to do the best to manage the situation and to cope with the changes that a disabling illness incurred. This was not just about protecting the partner or the marriage but also involved protecting oneself from the vulnerability that would be experienced if the relationship became fundamentally disrupted.

One of the most common responses when talking about how new roles that may be defined as caring were taken on was that 'it just happened'. At one level, this may be read to imply passivity or an absence of choice in taking on what would often be difficult or complex additional workloads. At another level, it marked the construction of additional caring in terms of the predominant ideology of marriage which reinforces the notion of caring for a spouse as an implicit obligation. Importantly, too, it was also frequently reinforced by motivations that emphasised the importance of maintaining continuity in a relationship which had been sustained for decades. The process by which motivations are translated into actual helping or assisting behaviour seemed to rely on the presence and interaction of a range of factors. My analysis of narratives suggested that four factors were central: choice, ability, being prepared and willingness to provide or receive care and support. I review, here, how these factors influenced motivation in providing care and support.

Mrs Blake, for example, described her marriage as an unhappy relationship characterised by disagreements, isolation and separateness. When Mr Blake became ill, Mrs Blake took on new and additional work, including providing physical, personal and supervisory care to him:

> I mean, he needs help and I'm here and there is only myself to do it. I have to do it and I have to keep going. It's strength of character I think because I don't think a lot of people would keep going. I think they'd say, well I've reached the end of my tether, you'll have to go.
>
> (Mrs Blake)

Mrs Blake was physically able to undertake the care work involved and, although in many ways unwilling to do it, felt she had little or no choice. Her lack of choice was reinforced by anxieties about her financial dependence upon her husband and a concern that she would not be able to afford to live if her husband moved into care. Mrs Blake identified her main motivation for caring for her spouse as marital duty and obligation. Later on, despite remaining physically able to assist her husband, Mrs Blake reached a point when she no longer felt willing to do it, and her earlier feeling that she had no choice had clearly changed. This had been influenced, to a large extent, by the couple's increasingly confrontational relationship, during which Mr Blake had responded with violence. Mr Blake was admitted to a residential home on a permanent basis and this was seen by Mrs Blake as the unhappy culmination of her long-standing unhappy marriage.

By contrast, Mr and Mrs Tompson identified themselves as having a close and happy marriage. As there was a significant range of caring tasks that Mr Tompson was unable to manage because of his own mobility difficulties, he arranged for others to do what he could not do. Mrs Tompson was, on the one hand, willing for her husband to be involved in her care but, in so doing, it served as a daily reminder to her of the change in herself as a competent and independent woman whose identity was closely tied in with a lifetime of providing for her husband and family. Mr Tompson was helping his wife physically in three main areas. In each area, Mrs Tompson praised her husband for his fortitude, but juxtaposed this with narrative which highlighted her own loss of skill and independence following her stroke and her husband's limited abilities in taking over these roles. In these examples, she talks about food preparation and mealtimes:

> Yes we shared everything. I mean a baking day my husband would be delighted to sample everything I cooked. With Yorkshire puddings and so on, you get into the habit, and I do think my husband is as fit as he is because he's had good home cooking. He's had it all his life.
> … since I've been ill my husband has taken over a lot. Whereas

before I'd taken over everything. And I find now the least little thing irritates him and he gets in a temper which I can't understand. You know he came to me with 'I can't find a frying pan anywhere'...I said 'we've four frying pans and one omelette pan. Surely you can find one.' Well he got so agitated. Now that I cannot understand.

In various ways, Mrs Tompson found ways to retain some degree of continuity in relation to her experience of domestic expertise by finding other ways to manage a situation she saw as outside her husband's capabilities. For example:

Well, I'm finding...you see I always used to do a lot of cooking. My husband has a big appetite and always appreciated my cooking. I can't do anything now. That worries me. The meals worry me. Now I've just been looking at the Voluntary Service for meals and I've been weighing up the cost. It's £1.70 for a main course. Now, I've been thinking to have those meals for two of us it's costing £20.00 a week for midday meals and I've been working out, could we do it cheaper than that?

Mr Tompson described looking after his wife as a positive choice, and he was willing to do all he could in order for them to remain together. In reality, he was unpractised at the tasks he would be required to do for his wife:

I observed her in hospital and how they put her in the chair and everything else, they always put the brakes on and that sort of thing. Cos I thought to myself I should have to do this myself if she ever comes home. So I did quite as much as I could in there, and when they knew we were coming home together they helped me as well. They gave me several tips on things I could do just by telling me. So I got along very well with that.

(Mr Tompson)

Providing personal and intimate care, as in the case of Mr and Mrs Dengate, provides an example of how choice, ability, being prepared and willing to provide or receive care and support can change over time. At the first interview, Mr and Mrs Dengate showed how they had managed the transition towards an amended role involving Mrs Dengate's bathing. This narrative was set in a context of reciprocity and was an example of negotiation. They both spoke about the importance of mutuality in assisting the other, and they spoke of satisfaction in achieving a resolution to Mrs Dengate's care need. Their solutions were in line with a key theme in their marital identity which was, in turn, powerfully reinforced by Mr Dengate's sense of self. Mr Dengate was a police officer and had also had experience of providing care to other family members. The whole idea of 'looking after your own' and 'finding one's own solutions' was an important relationship continuity. Mrs Dengate describes how they managed:

M:	How did you sort that out...did it just...
Mrs Dengate:	It just happened. He was the natural person to do it.
M:	Yes...did you ever talk about it?
Mrs Dengate:	No, not really.
M:	So, um, the first time John washed you...
Mrs Dengate	Well I do like to always feel clean and I can't bath... Saturday or Sunday is big wash day.
M:	Top to bottom?
Mrs Dengate:	Well I do down you know...
M:	You do your own bits...
Mrs Dengate:	I do my bits and pieces. Neither I nor John have ever said anything about it.
M:	You just know what you're doing.
Mrs Dengate:	Yes, I'll say...I've done as far as my waist and I'll leave my tummy to you. I'll go down to my knees and do the rest of my legs as we get to them so we never made that an issue.

At our follow-up contact, there had been significant changes in Mrs Dengate's health, and both were struggling to manage the joint reorganisation strategy that they had originally embarked upon. Mr Dengate was feeling increasingly ambivalent in terms of how prepared and willing he was to help his wife with personal care. In this extract, he explains these difficulties and emphasises a number of issues, including questioning his ability as a man to provide the care his wife needed:

It got so that she just refused to co-operate. We could have gone on with the same but I wasn't getting anywhere and it was taking me two hours so I got in touch with the DHSS...[social services] The girls [home care] come and dress her and she's down here finished all right. I still go up at the weekends. I'm not particularly a ladies' man, I do my best, but it's a job for me to get tights and that on, quite a job. Because don't forget, I've got to hold her with one hand and I've got to do everything with one hand. Well every morning that I got to do it, I get these tights on, pants on get her skirt on and she says I want a wee and I got to take it all back down again...

(Mr Dengate)

This example highlights that being willing and able to extend or receive help to a partner in managing one transition does not automatically follow into another area. This example demonstrates how a change in the balance of exchanges and availability of satisfactions in providing assistance can influence the ability to transfer support to other, more complex, tasks when rewards become more sparse (for example Ungerson, 1987). Together, these illustrations show how motivational states can ebb and flow over time in relation to the nature of the transitions that the couple are required to manage or reorganise.

The dynamic nature of care-giving tasks

The care-giving literature focuses significantly on cross-sectional approaches and, as a result, changes in care-giving roles are not easy to track over time. In my own study, the follow-up interviews with participants 6 months after initial contact revealed that the nature of care-giving often changed substantially over relatively short time periods. Within the reorganisation framework used in my analysis of narratives, changes are informed by the presence or absence of other disrupters (for example changes in health and well-being of either partner; changes in the provision of formal services) that may impede or have an impact on reorganisation attempts. Even within a relatively short follow-up period, it was possible to see considerable change in the way that couples had reorganised roles and responsibilities. For some participants, reorganisation attempts during the intervening period had involved using increasing levels of formal support. Partners who had been providing support were no longer able to maintain it or felt unable or unwilling to take on new roles and tasks. By our second contact, Mrs Hockney, for example, had relinquished many of the direct care tasks she undertook as she was no longer able to cope with the workload in terms of her own health and ability to tolerate her experience of stress and strain. She also experienced her marriage as having long-standing and unresolved difficulties and the impact of Mr Hockney's illness on the balance of exchange created fundamental difficulties for her in sustaining the level of care that she was expected to provide.

By the time I contacted the couple again to ask if I might visit for a follow-up interview, Mr Hockney had moved into a nursing home. Further reorganisation attempts at home were not tried, as Mrs Hockney had reached the end of her ability to keep going. Ultimately, Mr Blake and Mr Jenkins also moved into nursing care for similar reasons.

Mrs Blake described a marriage where caring had become such a feature of life that, in her experience, her marriage relationship had become subsumed by the caring relationship. Other women who defined their relationships as happy, satisfying and enjoyable were absolutely committed to the idea that they would not be parted from their husbands – whether they were providing care and support or receiving it. Mrs Francis and Mrs Tompson, for example, both spoke about the joint agreement that they would move as a couple into a care home should the need arise. Mr Drake, too, was so completely unable to provide care and support to his wife (by his own assessment) that his own reorganisation attempts were abandoned within weeks of her diagnosis of dementia, and he decided that they would move together into a nursing home where she could receive appropriate 'care and attention'.

For other participants, roles did not change significantly between my initial contact and follow-up meetings, and this indicated an overall absence of disruptions and success in stabilising changeful situations. For these couples, this had been achieved through an ability to assimilate new reorganisation strategies into their existing roles and responsibilities and to develop competence and familiarity in the way that they were accomplished. Nevertheless, while stability might mean not having to relinquish roles on the part of the disabled partner, or take on new roles for the supportive spouse, it did mean that, for some partners, they were coping with heavy workloads and onerous management of day-to-day tasks. The emotional consequences and challenges of coping could still be significant.

Concluding discussion

The brief review of literature in this chapter confirms that, overwhelmingly, much existing research on long-term marriage and care-giving makes use of quantitative methodologies with cross-sectional designs. Taken together, they provide a significant knowledge base, but differences in the ways that terms such as caring, marital satisfaction and stress and burden have been operationalised make straightforward comparisons problematic.

In the broadest terms, my own study supports some of the main conclusions from reported research. For example, most of the women participants identified themselves as being happily married but had also demonstrated considerable tenacity, flexibility and fortitude in managing the challenges that were inevitably associated with a relationship lasting decades. This observation has to be set in the context of the cohort of women and men in the study who were profoundly influenced by social and cultural ideologies of power and influence in marriage relationships.

Moreover, although the emergence of caring relationships in the context of marriage has been examined, it has rarely been explored longitudinally or from the perspective of both partners in the relationship. My own research has found support for the importance of considering the context of the relationship in which caring takes place (Parker, 1993, 1994). The narratives of both partners provide important insights into the ways in which, for example, marriage biographies or identities were used as a backdrop in the maintenance, or reconstruction, of identity when the transitions created by disability threatened long-standing continuities. The issue of continuity was clearly very important, and Atchley's (1989) work on continuity theory was particularly relevant to the ways in which participants in my own study made sense of the transitions they faced. Looking at a process of transition from both partners' perspectives also brought into sharper focus the women and men who receive care, who, in the caring literature, remain essentially invisible. It highlights that women who were cared for by partners were not inevitably passive inactive bystanders. The women in my study continued to participate in their lives as much as they were able. Even when active participation was no longer an option, the women continued to have their lives shaped by the experience of managing transition and change, and this must not be overlooked in a discourse which focuses entirely on the 'caregiver'.

Marriage biographies that were assessed by women as being successful appeared to have an understandably higher baseline of mutuality, reciprocity and a perception of an appropriate balance of exchange (for example Parker, 1993). In this context, women participants, whether providing or receiving support and care, were able to continue to both use and identify relationship strengths and continuities which reinforced and affirmed important aspects of their marriage identities. A severe or persistent loss of reciprocity or balance of exchange caused by unhappy marriage histories or by long unrelenting caring created relationships at risk of becoming overwhelmed by the stress and strain of providing physical, emotional and practical care and support. This adds further support to the importance of formal agencies taking the time to understand the ways in which couples assess and construct their marriage relationships.

A longitudinal perspective, even over a short time period, confirmed that caring relationships are also dynamic and ever changing. They do not stand still, but alter in relation to the challenges that arise and to the motivations and abilities of partners to continue to reorganise and restructure solutions to them. Even when the women in the study were released from day-to-day care, they continued to have considerable caring responsibilities in terms of supporting their husbands who had moved into care.

A detailed look at the caring process also confirmed the variety of ways in which individuals defined and constructed their roles and responsibilities. These were undoubtedly influenced by gender and the ways in which responsibilities and power relationships were formed within long-term marriage. It was clear (and obvious) that the ways in which women constructed caring roles were fundamentally influenced by their marriage biographies and the normative expectations that they experienced in that context. But, there was considerable diversity, for example, among the women participants in terms of the way that they defined their roles and made sense of giving or receiving support.

This chapter set out to explore some aspects of a qualitative research project which examined long-term marriage relationships in the context of emerging chronic illness and disability. In so doing, it has challenged certain features associated with both marriage and caring for women in old age, emphasising, in particular, the variability with which women define and construct caring roles, the diverse and complex nature of caring and the wide range of marital biographies. These all fundamentally influence the way women shape and make sense of managing a time of transition and change brought on by their own or their spouse's illness or disability.

10 Women ageing

Changing policy, challenging practice

Judith Phillips and Miriam Bernard

If every day is an awakening, you will never grow old. You will just keep growing.

(Gail Sheehy, 1995: 429)

Introduction

This book has been about growing in our understanding of ageing, as it confronts women in general and ourselves in particular. The central chapters attempted to highlight the changing identities of women as they age while, at the same time, challenging a number of myths about women's roles in the home, at work and in education. Key themes in women's lives were reviewed by drawing on our own empirical work, from existing literature and research findings and from our practice experience in a variety of arenas.

This concluding chapter draws together two major strands: it reflects, first, on the content of the book and, second, on the process of writing the book. We outline policy and practice implications arising from each chapter and discuss these under five themes which we believe are important for informing future policy and practice. We argue that policy and practice is inherently gendered and built upon myths and stereotypes and suggest, instead, that they should recognise the changing contexts in which women live their lives; reflect women's diverse and multiple identities; give a voice to mid-life and older women; and focus more on women's abilities, on creating positive images and on having meaning and relevance at an individual level. This is followed by a discussion of potential research agendas and ways of researching older women's lives. This is necessary to understand the issues facing future cohorts, and is important to the design of appropriate policies and practices in the twenty-first century.

In writing the book, we have also matured as authors, through a process of collective writing, commenting, critiquing and sharing ideas. We documented our experiences of the process and, in so doing, have been able to begin to look at aspects of our own ageing and at some of our own blindspots. Writing collectively and reflexively provided an empowering and creative forum in which to work, as well as posing challenges. We therefore discuss both the frustrations and the fun in such an enterprise. Finally, we offer a comment on the situation of critical feminist gerontology in the UK, and assess the contribution of this book to wider debates in gerontology.

Changing policy, challenging practice

Given the increasing number of ageing women in the population and the concomitant effects that this has on the demographics of work, education and care, analyses presented in these chapters are of importance to policy-makers and practitioners, particularly those who work with or formulate policy for older people. Here, we examine common issues for policy-makers and practitioners, emphasising five key themes or messages arising from the discussions in previous chapters:

* policies and practices are not gender neutral;
* the policy context and the practice response is subject to change;
* policy and practice should not be built on stereotypes and myths but should recognise women's changing identities and images;
* policy-making and practice arenas should give ageing women a voice;
* policy and practice should focus on abilities and associated positive images and should have meaning and relevance to individuals.

First, *policies and practices are not gender neutral*, as is so often portrayed in much of the existing literature. The traditional models of work, referred to, for example, in Chapters 2, 3 and 9, are based on a male breadwinner image and fail to take account of the new world of work where women play an increasingly important role. Moving from masculine models of work to models embracing flexibility and part-time work is necessary if we are more accurately to reflect and estimate women's contributions to the labour market. Women's unpaid work also needs to be urgently re-evaluated.

In Chapter 2, Julie Skucha and Miriam Bernard also highlighted the broader issue of gendered work cultures. Here, there is a need for more extensive research into how employers respond to women and men in the workplace, and how and what models can be introduced without reinforcing gender stereotypes and sex segregation. Traditionally, occupational welfare benefits served to maintain the gendered division of labour (Sara Arber and Jay Ginn 1993), but flexible working, for example, may in fact be detrimental to women in terms of their entitlement to occupational pensions. Similarly, further research needs to address attitudes at all levels within organisations in relation to existing stereotypes and to caring in general. As Judith Phillips shows in Chapter 3, it is important to recognise men's involvement in caring so that caring is not viewed solely as a women's problem, nor does it become just women who are seen as having a problem with caring.

Caring is also a crucial issue in relation to long-term marriage and disability. Mo Ray, in Chapter 9, drew our attention to the diversity of experiences and definitions of caring across gender, making a simple dichotomy between men and women problematic. A gendered approach to caring and working across the adult life-course is therefore vital if we are to understand more fully how these intersect with ageing and if we are to develop policy and practice appropriately.

Second, *the policy context and the consequent practice response is subject to continual change* and, indeed, contradictions. In our view, much more account must be taken of the changing needs of mid-life and older women. The demographic imperative brings this into sharp focus, and successive cohorts of women will experience very different collective and individual life histories which may well include a rising incidence of divorce and remarriage. More women will be entering mid- and later life alone or as part of 'reconstituted' families. Consequently, future social policy is likely to be increasingly concerned with issues such as the vulnerabilities of lone women accessing resources and intergenerational transfers between step-families.

Moreover, the continued reorganisation of health and social welfare services in the UK will also have profound implications for women in mid- and later life. The linking together of public, voluntary and private care systems is important in the development of initiatives, but further research is required on how this can most effectively be achieved. In the last two decades, there has been overwhelming policy attention on the role of women as carers. As we enter the twenty-first century, a National Strategy for Carers (Her Majesty's Government, 1999) sets out three strategic elements: around information, support and care. It recognises that women have multiple identities, not only participating in caring roles (often across long distances) but also contributing to society as employees. Elder care is now seen as an important issue to be addressed by employers and policy-makers, with interventions based around policies relating to leave, part-time work, flexi-time and career breaks. Different images of women carers are therefore beginning to be reflected in policy and strategy. However, one key question that remains unanswered from policy initiatives or from our own research on women's work (see Chapters 2, 3 and 9) is exactly what kinds of public services and supports do women find most helpful to keep them in employment? Alongside this, it is also vital to know under what conditions external help and support becomes acceptable to women, and how we can improve the perception of public sector welfare – particularly the view of residential care – if carers are to be adequately assisted.

Likewise, the world of education policy and practice is also changing rapidly. In Chapter 6, Patsy Marshall highlighted the potential for lifelong learning in the twenty-first century; a potential which in theory at least will increase as traditional work and retirement boundaries breakdown. However, by discontinuing grants for first-time undergraduates and excluding people aged 54 plus from the Student Loan Scheme, a likely future outcome is that many mid-life and older women will in fact be denied the opportunities to realise the benefits of the stereotypical third-age lifestyle much espoused by current policy-makers.

The third central message of this book is therefore that *policy and practice should not be built on stereotypes and myths*. Rather, it should recognise and acknowledge women's changing identities and diverse images and experiences. Pat Chambers highlighted this in her chapter on widowhood (Chapter 8), drawing attention to the need to challenge and reframe the current policy conception of widows as lonely and in need of care, income and support. While not denying that this view reflects the experiences of some women, it is only a partial and incomplete image of widowhood. Many of Pat Chambers's respondents did not in fact see widowhood as a period of decline, but embraced it as another phase in their lives with opportunities for continuing change and development. We hope that by using such examples throughout the central chapters of this book we have challenged some of the uniform stereotypes so often presented in policy forums and practices.

Our fourth theme concerns the need to *give ageing women a voice in policy-making and in practice arenas*. Increasingly, the voices of ageing women are being heard through recent initiatives, such as the Better Government for Older People programme. It is to be hoped that such developments will enable older women to exert a much greater influence than previously on policies and practices concerned with important and closely related areas, including health, housing, work, education, local government services, transport, crime and many other issues affecting women's lives.

For us, policies and practices concerning women's health are areas which still need much attention, despite the inroads made by the women's health movement over the last few decades. Gillian Granville (Chapter 5) argues that health policy agendas have yet to understand fully the needs of women at mid-life. In particular, this must include opportunities for ageing women to make sense of their changing bodies without it being regarded as automatically requiring treatment. Practitioners, both in health and in social welfare agencies, therefore need to listen to mid-life and older women, giving them opportunities to talk about their experiences and define their own concerns rather than having them constructed by others.

Mo Ray too (see Chapter 9) highlights the importance of listening to the voices of older women. In her case, this concerns the ways in which social work assessments need to take account of the impact of joint and individual biographies in order to understand how this kind of long-term relationship has an impact on caring and other activities in late old age. Formal agencies must take time to understand the ways in which couples assess and construct their marriage relationship if caring is to be fully understood and properly supported.

Our fifth and final theme therefore concerns the ways in which listening to the voices of mid-life and older women should also help to ensure that *policy and practice focuses more on older women's abilities*. In so doing, this should in turn help contribute to more positive images as well as having meaning and relevance to individuals. The central chapters have illustrated some of the diversity in women's lives: their experiences and reflections between, and within, different cohorts. Policy and practice, however, do not always recognise or take account of such diversity. For example, the chapters by Linda Machin and Pat Chambers show just how wide a range of reactions and responses exist to bereavement and grief as an acute state or as a process of being bereaved. Pat Chambers's respondents convey a different and somewhat more positive picture than that which emerges from Linda Machin's study in which mid-life and older women, often years after their husband's death, sought out counselling. However, Linda Machin importantly calls attention to the need to acknowledge that women have a wide range of reactions to bereavement, most of which can be regarded as non-pathological. It is the role of the counsellor to hear and take note of the individual voice, but the role of policy-makers and practitioners to ensure that whatever strategies are developed they have meaning to individuals.

Furthermore, as Mo Ray's research highlights (see Chapter 9), the active, complex and persistent attempts that long-married couples make to manage difficult situations should not be undermined by formal agencies with reductionist assessment approaches, which are ultimately tests for eligibility. True assessment of need should explore and build upon the strengths, abilities and resources in people's biographies.

We also need to recognise, as Gillian Granville has shown in her chapter about the menopause (Chapter 5), that there are other ways to approach and understand aspects of women's lives which move us away from decremental and negative images of what ageing is like for women. Alongside the prevailing negative imagery, ageing also brings opportunities and strengths which we need to acknowledge and work with. Moreover, as Val Harding

Davies and Miriam Bernard argue (see Chapter 4), establishing more positive images will only come about if we engage in discussion and debate with mid-life and older women instead of perpetuating an 'us' and 'them' mentality.

Women researching: reflections on method

In the introductory chapter, we briefly discussed the variety of methods used in our own research studies. These methods reflect our desire to move away from the 'add women and stir' approach of much earlier work while, at the same time, addressing issues central to the lives of mid-life and older women. Our work has used both qualitative and quantitative approaches together with a recognition that our own concerns and biographies will inevitably influence what we study, how we study it and how we interpret our data. Reflecting on the methods we have adopted, we draw from this a number of points which we believe are worthy of further development.

First, several chapters have called for a longitudinal perspective to be adopted in future research. Such an approach would better illustrate the continuities in women's lives, as well as the diversity of their experience and their abilities. Our current, and largely cross-sectional approaches, tell us little, for example, about the entrances and exits that women experience in relation to the workplace over the course of their lives or about what would help them juggle work and family life or assist them in lifelong learning. As Mo Ray argues (see Chapter 9), longitudinal approaches can help to illustrate the ways in which continuities are used to construct current identities, as well as explaining the ways in which strategies for managing change are used. In research terms, the complexity and diversity of the way that caring roles are defined and are dynamic make the overwhelming focus on cross-sectional quantitative study somewhat problematic.

Second, the complexity and diversity of women's lives needs to be overtly linked into a life-course perspective if women are to benefit from developing policies and practices. Closely related to this is the use of narrative and biography as research tools for bringing the voices of mid-life and older women to the forefront. By adopting an approach which acknowledges individual biography and its influences on resources, roles and relationships, we can begin the process of better integrating research findings into theory building (Arber and Ginn, 1995; Bury, 1995). At the same time, this should also offer insights of value to practitioners working with still marginalised groups of mid-life and older women (Marie Mills, 1999).

Finally, there is also scope in the future to engage in a much more interactive research process with respondents themselves. This would extend not simply to a greater focus on mid-life and older women as subjects rather than objects of research but would also engage them in the process, reporting and writing of research. To date, there is comparatively little research of this kind, although some examples have been written up and published (see, for example, Patricia Thornton and Rosemary Tozer, 1995).

Women writing: reflections on the collaborative process

This book has also been about the process of ageing itself: a journey of growing older. For all of us, it has been a journey of discovery – into that uncharted territory of collaborative writing and reflection. A journey requires planning: it involves a destination, pace, navigational aides and signposts, and an idea of distance, gradient and terrain. It will also be experienced differently by each traveller. It draws on perceptions, past experiences and anticipation, excitement and trepidation. It is never straightforward: you can lose your way, take the wrong turning or need to turn back and ask for directions. All of these aspects have been experienced during the writing of this book.

The group first came together to talk about the possibilities of a collaborative project in 1995. Through the life of the group, however, there were changes both in focus and membership. Initially, the project was to encompass women at different phases across the entire adult life-course. However, job changes and illness resulted in some members leaving the group and new members joining. This in turn led to a sharper focus for the book and it evolved into a project concerned primarily with the experiences of mid-life and older women.

Writing the book has been essentially an exercise in trust. For some of us, this was the first experience of writing for publication and of writing collaboratively. Over time, as we got to know each other better, we all grew in confidence and were able to share our material and to challenge each other. Sharing raw versions of chapters and critiquing chapters that we have worked on for considerable periods can be a nerve-racking experience. We all learnt, though, to share our writing and to give and receive feedback constructively and sensitively. Sometimes, we had to be strong enough to make less than positive comments about the work of colleagues, and we all learnt how to receive and use criticism in a positive way. An exercise in 'patience, growing through a painful process' was how one of us described the experience.

Devising agreed and complementary formats and structures for the central chapters was a useful device, especially for 'new' authors. As the book evolved, growing familiarity with the content of one another's developing chapters also helped to inform our own chapters. Rather than writing a chapter in isolation, being able to read, comment, develop and suggest ideas for other chapters was a satisfying experience. The pleasure of meeting up periodically with other women in a collective enterprise, sharing ideas, feelings and nice food as well as the hard work made the process fun. Without exception, we all felt that it was a supportive and enjoyable experience and that having ownership of the book through such collaboration was valuable.

Not surprisingly, our professional as well as personal lives had an impact on the process – time was a key issue. Difficulties of writing something coherent when time-scales were pressing created particular tensions. Those of us who are practitioners and academics found the project squeezed into late-night work. Frustration about the time that the process took also came to the surface, especially when we talked too much about the chapters rather than wrote. For some of us, this possibly reflected a lack of confidence in ourselves to get going with the writing. But, for all of us, the process of sharing was supportive, particularly during times when a number of personal changes and crises occurred. Nor did these inevitable difficulties hamper us in our collective reflection on each chapter and, overall, we feel strengthened by the exercise.

Women ageing: reflections on our own ageing

Ruth Ray, in her address to the Gerontological Society of America in November 1999, claims that 'to empower others through our research and practice, we must first know and empower ourselves. It is a feminist responsibility to become more self-conscious, self-reflexive, and self-critical.'

A feature which shaped the process of our writing, but which is not made explicit in each chapter, is the location and self-consciousness of each writer: although we may reveal our ideas about an issue, we do not reveal our innermost thoughts about the impact that the writing and thinking has had on us as ageing women ourselves. Perhaps we have not gone far enough? In an attempt to rectify this, we convened a group meeting towards the end of the writing, specifically to reflect on our own ageing and the impact the book had had so far on our own thoughts and behaviour.

We are at different points in the journey of ageing ourselves: for some of us, mid-life is a new experience, whereas for others the challenges of biological ageing have already come into view, along with the opportunities presented through retirement and the relinquishing of parental roles. For all of us though, later life experiences could only be considered and anticipated. Yet, many of the themes discussed in the book have been experienced by us first hand. During the writing, three of us lost a parent after prolonged illness and several of us changed jobs or undertook courses of further study. Experiencing menopause, caring for frail older parents, supporting partners going through redundancy and retirement also mirror the experiences of the women described in the central chapters.

What impact then did the book have on our understanding of our own ageing? For all of us, it raised some uncomfortable issues, particularly the difficulties in contemplating caring on a long-term basis for a sick partner or, even worse, in one person's experience, being cared for long term by her husband. Without doubt, writing the book has also made us all more conscious of our own feelings of getting older: we found ourselves continually making comparisons between the text and our own circumstances. The thought of our bodies being less reliable heightened our awareness of the accumulation of losses that take place as we move through the life-course. Although regarded as one of the negatives of ageing, we considered this to be one of things that make us the women that we are. We all felt that we had to take care of ourselves by taking exercise and eating healthily. Ageing just sharpens the necessity of these.

Our positions in a social network was an area of lively discussion. Some of us felt we were 'notching up a generation' following the death of parents. One of us voiced this as coming to terms with being 'at the top of the tree', with both parents having died, having no siblings and no very close family. Fears of loneliness in later life and perceiving oneself as an 'orphan' were the downside. There was also a temptation to reject or not acknowledge our own ageing and position in the family in this way, and issues around bereavement and ageing drew painful parallels for many of us. There were also inconsistencies and ambivalences about our own ageing. One of us admitted to buying a pot of 'age-defying cream' and to having a fear of her hair being perceived as frumpish so had it cut regularly. Wearing glasses was another area of ambivalence and a distinctive marker of age for some. We recognised that although we may feel all right about physically ageing we still try to take control of it and may in fact be hiding our ageing from ourselves and others.

The book has also led us to reflect on how we might cope with issues beyond our present experience. In coping with widowhood, one of us hoped that she would be publicly brave, perhaps privately counting the losses but seeing the potential for growth as noted in Pat Chambers's chapter (Chapter 8). There were also positive aspects and opportunities associated with the ageing process: no longer having to juggle with bits of life; being able to serve our own needs; being more self-confident; recognising the things we cannot do; being more willing and able to forgive ourselves; learning to be more accepting; and being able to decide things for oneself rather than being subject to the rules and regulations of the systems and institutions that employ us.

Finally, writing this book has also helped us, as academics, to be more aware of how we present some of the issues to our students. We must be careful that academic insights are not seen as objective but are personal to us too. We are constantly schooled not to make these connections, and are at pains not to let our own experiences of ageing have an impact on our gerontological, social work or counselling teaching. Sharing in such a way is viewed as too risky and does not square with (masculine) notions of academic rigour. Our experience suggests that this is an academic blind spot and that critical self-reflection and analysis has a part to play in both what and how we teach and research.

Conclusion: where to now?

We don't just suddenly age: we slowly move towards old age, passing biological and social signposts such as the menopause and retirement. We bring with us on the journey baggage from the past and identities shaped by earlier periods in life. Attitudes, aspirations and expectations develop and shape our responses as we age, whether it be in the realm of care, health, work or education. Loss is a constant and continual experience, without which we cannot go on. Ageing also intersects with the social, economic and political developments which shape the terrain and a wide diversity of experience is the inevitable result.

In this book, we have adopted a critical feminist life-course perspective to take a snapshot of ageing women at the start of the twenty-first century. This approach has been essential to the thinking and development of the book and builds on earlier work (Sara Arber and Jay Ginn, 1991, 1995; Miriam Bernard and Kathy Meade, 1993). In Chapters 5 and 8, the authors adopted an overtly feminist approach, while others have drawn on a range of theories and methods not necessarily described as feminist but nevertheless focused on women's lives and women's identities. In line with a feminist approach, we were also conscious of the need to make women academics more visible in the literature. Thus, readers will also be aware that we have referenced female authors differently from male authors – putting in their first and second names when they are initially cited in each chapter.

In conclusion then, what does this say in relation to the state of critical feminist gerontology in the UK; what claims can the book make in contributing to the field and where do we go from here?

We have attempted in this book to go beyond pure description of women's lives and to engage in an analysis of key issues from a variety of viewpoints. Gerontology in the UK has been enriched by feminist perspectives which have not only begun to look critically at the experience of growing old, but have also challenged traditional assumptions about older and ageing women. We have also looked at issues such as identity from a life-course perspective, recognising the potential for change throughout life. Although we have not overtly applied a post-modernist perspective throughout our work, what we have discussed is essentially the post-modern feminist life-course: looking at diversity, difference and sites of oppression in health and paid work, as well as challenging accepted myths about caring, working, education and responses to bereavement and widowhood. In this sense, we have integrated age and gender with other dimensions of oppression, while recognising the importance of the diverse experience of ageing and old age itself.

Many of the chapters have addressed the breakdown in the traditional stages of the life-course – education, marriage, work, retirement and bereavement – which no longer occur in a linear process and are no longer (if they ever were) gender neutral. Growing older is not a straightforward journey to a fixed destination, but has numerous routes with various experiences which overlap and intersect. Mid- and later life is not unidimensional, as our reflections highlight, with several of the themes in the book running parallel in women's lives: work and care; bereavement and leisure; education and retirement. We have also highlighted both the diversity and the continuity within cohorts. Post-modern feminism seeks to be inclusive and we have also attempted in some of our methodologies to engage in empirical reflection with older women themselves.

However, our conclusions about ageing are our own, drawn from individual biases and preconceptions and may not in fact reflect the perceptions of older women themselves. Nor do we claim to have represented the complete range of diverse experiences of women. We have not, for example, addressed to any great extent the experiences of women of race and colour, cultural differences, bisexual or lesbian women or of women in very late old age or in different living environments. We recognise the limitations of the book and that it is only making visible the lives of certain mid-life and older women.

Gerontology as a subject is also on a journey, moving from its concentration on a destination, old age, to a more flexible and inclusive investigation of the journey of ageing through mid- and into later life. Although our final destination in this process has been reached, and the book is written and published, it has been a journey for all of us, personally and professionally, as academics and practitioners, as daughters, wives and mothers. What we have yet to do is to further this approach by undertaking practical project work, by disseminating our ideas and findings more widely and, most importantly, by engaging older women from a wide variety of backgrounds in a critical commentary of our work. Such are the new challenges ahead for us as ageing women.

Bibliography

Achenbaum, W.A. (1997) 'Critical gerontology', in A. Jamieson, S. Harper and C. Victor (eds) *Critical Approaches to Ageing and Later Life*, Buckingham: Open University Press.

Achenbaum, W.A. and Levin, J.S. (1989) 'What does *gerontology* mean?', *The Gerontologist* 29, 3: 393–400.

Acker, S. (1980) 'Women, the other academics', in Equal Opportunities Commission *Equal Opportunities in Higher Education*, Report of an EOC/SRHE Conference at Manchester Polytechnic, Manchester: Equal Opportunities Commission.

Addison, G. (1985) *Now the War is Over, A Social History of Britain 1945–51*, London: The British Broadcasting Corporation.

Adelman, M. (1986) *Long Time Passing: Lives of Older Lesbians*, Boston: Aylison Publications.

Ade-Ridder, L. and Brubaker, T. (1988) 'Expected and reported divisions of responsibility of household tasks among older wives in two residential settings', *Journal of Consumer Studies and Home Economics* 12: 59–70.

Adkins, L. and Lury, C. (1992) 'Gender and the labour market: old theory for new?', in H. Hinds *et al*. (eds) *Working Out: New Directions in Women's Studies*, London: Falmer Press.

Adlersberg, M. and Thorne, S. (1992) 'Emerging from the chrysalis', *Journal of Gerontological Nursing* 6: 4–8.

Age Concern (1998) *Factsheet*, London: Age Concern England.

Alford-Cooper, F. (1998) *For Keeps: Marriages That Last A Lifetime*. New York: M.E. Sharpe.

Allen, K. (1989) *Single Women/Family Ties: Life Histories of Older Women*, Newbury Park, CA: Sage.

Althusser, L. (1971) 'Ideology and ideological state apparatuses', in L. Althusser (ed.) *Lenin and Philosophy and Other Essays*, London: New Left Books.

Anderson, K., Armitage, S., Jack, D., Wittner, J. (1987) 'Beginning where we are: feminist methodology in oral history', *Oral History Review* 57: 103–27.

Andrews, M. (1999) 'The seductiveness of agelessness', *Ageing and Society* 19, 3: 301–18.

Antonucci, T. (1985) 'Personal characteristics, social support and social behaviour', in R.H. Binstock and E. Shanas (eds) *Handbook of Aging and Social Sciences*, New York: Van Nostrand Reinhold.

Apter, T. (1995) *Secret Paths: Women in the New Mid-life*, New York: W.W. Norton.
——(1996) 'Paths of development for mid-life women', *Feminism and Psychology* 6, 4: 557–62.
Arber, S. and Ginn, J. (1991) *Gender and Later Life – A Sociological Analysis of Resources and Constraints*, London: Sage.
——(1993) 'Class, caring and the lifecourse' in S. Arber and M. Evandrou (eds) *Ageing, Independence and the Life Course*, London: Jessica Kingsley.
——(eds) (1995) *Connecting Gender and Ageing: a Sociological Approach*, Buckingham: Open University Press.
Arling, G. (1976) 'The elderly widow and her family, neighbours and friends', *Journal of Marriage and the Family* November: 757–68.
Askham, J. (1994) 'Marriage relationships of older people', *Reviews in Clinical Gerontology* 4, 3: 261–8.
——(1995) 'The married lives of older people', in S. Arber and J. Ginn (eds) *Connecting Gender and Ageing: a Sociological Approach*, Buckingham: Open University Press.
Askham, J., Grundy, E. and Tinker, A. (1992) *Caring: The Importance of Third Age Carers*. Research paper no. 6. Carnegie Inquiry into the Third Age. Dunfermline: The Carnegie Trust.
Atchley, R.C. (1975) 'Dimensions of widowhood in later life', *The Gerontologist* 15: 176–8.
——(1989) 'A continuity theory of normal aging', *The Gerontologist* 29, 2: 183–90.
——(1992) 'Retirement and marital satisfaction', in M. Szinovacz, D. Ekerdt and B. Vinick (eds) *Families and Retirement*, Thousand Oaks, CA: Sage.
——(1993) 'Continuity theory and the evolution of activity in later adulthood', in J.R. Kelly (ed.) *Activity and Aging, Staying Involved in Later Life*, London: Sage.
Attig, T. (1996) *How We Grieve: Relearning the World*. New York: Oxford University Press.
Babchuk, N. and Anderson, T.B. (1989) 'Older widows and married women, their intimates and their confidantes', *International Journal of Ageing and Human Development* 7: 67–86.
Bankoff, E. (1983) 'Social support and adaptation to widowhood', *Journal of Marriage and the Family*, November: 827–39.
Bartholomew, K. (1990) 'Avoidance of intimacy: an attachment perspective', *Journal of Social and Personal Relationships*, 7: 147–78.
Barusch, A. and Spaid, W. (1989) 'Gender differences in caregiving: why do wives report greater burden?', *The Gerontologist* 29, 5: 667–75.
Beasley, C. (1999) *What is Feminism?* London: Sage Publications.
de Beauvoir, S. (1969) *A Very Easy Death,* London: Penguin.
Belcher, I. (1999) 'All that glitters…', *Observer Magazine* 7 November: 42–8.
Berger, G. (1999) *Menopause and Culture*, London: Pluto Press.
Bergkvist, I., Adami, H.-O., Persson, I., Hoover, R. and Schairer, C. (1989) 'The risk of breast cancer after oestrogen's and oestrogen/progestin replacement', *New England Journal of Medicine* 321: 293–7.

Bernard, M. (1998) 'Backs to the future? Reflections on women, ageing and nursing', *Journal of Advanced Nursing* 27: 633–40.

Bernard, M. and Meade, K. (eds) (1993a) *Women Come of Age – Perspectives on the Lives of Older Women*, London: Edward Arnold.

——(1993b) 'Perspectives on the lives of older women', in M. Bernard and K. Meade (eds) *Women Come of Age – Perspectives on the Lives of Older Women*, London: Edward Arnold.

Bevan, C. and Gattuso, S. (1998) 'Emotional labour in aged care', unpublished paper presented at the Australian Association of Gerontology Conference, Melbourne, 1998.

Biggs, S. (1993) *Understanding Ageing: Images, Attitudes and Professional Practice*, Buckingham: Open University Press.

——(1997) 'Choosing not to be old? Masks, bodies and identity management in later life', *Ageing and Society* 17, 15: 553–70.

——(1999a) *The Mature Imagination: Dynamics and Identity in Mid-life and Beyond*, Buckingham: Open University Press.

——(1999b) 'The blurring of the lifecourse: narrative, memory and the question of authenticity', unpublished paper given at the Economic and Social Research Council (ESRC) seminar series 'Age and Identity', University of Keele, June.

Billington, R., Hockey, J. and Strawbridge, S. (1998) *Exploring Self and Society*. London: Macmillan.

Birren, J. (1996) 'Aging and biography', in J. Birren, G. Kenyon, J.E. Ruth, J.J.F. Schroots and T. Svensson (eds) *Explorations in Adult Development*, New York: Springer.

Blackburn, R.M. and Jarman, J. (1993) 'Changing inequalities in access to British universities', *Oxford Review of Education* 19, 2: 197–215.

Blau, Z. (1973) *Old Age in a Changing Society*, New York: Franklin Watts.

Blunkett, D. (1998) *The Learning Age, A Renaissance for a New Britain*. London: DfEE, The Stationery Office.

Boaz, A., Hayden, C. and Bernard, M. (1999) *Attitudes and Aspirations of Older People: A Review of the Literature*, London: Department of Social Security Research Series.

Boland, E. (1996) *Object Lessons: The Life of the Woman and the Poet in Our Time*, London: Vintage.

Bond, J., Coleman, P. and Peace, S. (eds) (1993) *Ageing in Society – An Introduction to Social Gerontology*, 2nd edn, London: Sage.

Bornat, J. (1993) 'Life experience', in M. Bernard and K. Meade (eds) *Women Come of Age – Perspectives on the Lives of Older Women*, London: Edward Arnold.

Bourdieu, P. (1977) 'Cultural reproduction and social reproduction', in J. Karabel and A.H. Halsey (eds) *Power and Ideology in Education*, New York: Oxford University Press.

Bowlby, J. (1980) *Attachment and Loss*. Vol. 1. *Attachment*, New York: Basic Books.

Bowles, S. and Gintis, H. (1976) *Schooling in Capitalist America*, London: Routledge and Kegan Paul.

Bowling, A. and Cartwright, A. (1982) *Life After A Death*, London: Tavistock Publishing.

Brannen, J. and Moss, P. (1991) *Mothers: Dual Earner Households after Maternity Leave*, London: Macmillan.

Brannen, J., Meszaras, G., Moss, P. and Poland, G. (1994) *Employment and Family Life: A Review of Research in the UK (1980–1994)*, London: Employment Department.

Braudy-Harris, P. (1993) 'The misunderstood caregiver? A qualitative study of male caregivers of Alzheimer's disease victims', *The Gerontologist* 33, 4: 551–6.

Brody, E. (1990) *Women in the Middle: Their Parent-Care Years,* New York: Springer Publishing Company.

Browne, C.V. (1998) *Women, Feminism and Aging*, New York: Springer Series: Focus on Women.

Brubaker, T. (1985) 'Responsibility for household tasks: a look at Golden Anniversary couples aged 75 years and older', in W. Peterson and J. Quadagno (eds) *Social Bonds in Later Life*, Newbury Park, CA: Sage.

——(1990) 'Families in later life: a burgeoning research area', *Journal of Marriage and the Family* 5: 959–81.

Brubaker, T. and Ade-Ridder, L. (1986) 'Husbands' responsibility for household tasks in older marriages: does living situation make a difference?', in R. Lewis and E. Salt (eds) *Men in Families*, Newbury Park, CA: Sage.

Brubaker, T. and Hennon, C.B. (1982) 'Responsibility for household tasks: comparing dual earner and dual retired marriages', in M. Szinovacz (ed.) *Women's Retirement: Policy Implications of Recent Research*, Newbury Park, CA: Sage.

Buck, N. Gershuny, J. Rose, D. and Scott, J. (1994) *Changing Households. The British Household Panel Survey, 1990–1992.* Essex: Economic and Social Research Council (ESRC) Research Centre on Micro-social Change.

Burr, V. (1995) *An Introduction to Social Constructionism,* London: Routledge,

Bury, M. (1995) 'Ageing, gender and sociological theory', in S. Arber and J. Ginn (eds) *Connecting Gender and Ageing: a Sociological Approach*, Buckingham: Open University Press.

Butler, J. (1990) *Gender Trouble*, New York: Routledge.

Butler, R.N. (1980) 'Ageism: a foreword', *Journal of Social Issues* 36, 2: 8–11.

Bytheway, B. (1997) 'Talking about age: the theoretical basis of social gerontology', in A. Jamieson, S. Harper and C. Victor (eds) *Critical Approaches to Ageing and Later Life*, Buckingham: Open University Press.

Bytheway, B. and Johnson, J. (1990) 'On defining ageism', *Critical Social Policy* 27: 27–39.

Calasanti, T. (1999) 'Feminism and gerontology: not just for women', *Hallym International Journal of Aging* 1: 44–56.

Calasanti, T.M. and Zajicek, A.M. (1993) 'A socialist–feminist approach to aging: embracing diversity', *Journal of Aging Studies* 7, 2: 117–31.

Cannon, C. (ed.) (2000) *Our Grandmothers, Our Mothers, Ourselves*, London: Ogomos.

Caraway, N. (1991) *Segregated Sisterhood: Racism and the Politics of American Feminism*, Knoxville, TN: University of Tennessee Press.

Carlton, S. and Soulsby, J. (1999) *Learning to Grow Older and Bolder*, Leicester: National Institute of Adult and Continuing Education.

Carolan, M. (1994) 'Beyond deficiency: broadening the view of menopause', *The Journal of Applied Gerontology* 13, 2: 193–205.

Chambers, P. (1994) 'A biographical approach to widowhood' *Generations Review* 4, 3: 8–12.

——(1998) 'Involving older women in the research process', *Generations Review* 8, 4: 6–8.

Chirawatkul, S. and Manderson, L. (1994) 'Perceptions of menopause in Northeast Thailand: contested meaning and practice', *Social Science and Medicine* 39: 1545–54.

Cleiren, M. (1991) *Bereavement and Adaptation,* Washington: Hemisphere Publishing.

Clennell, S. *et al.* (eds) (1987) *Older Students in Adult Education*, Buckingham: The Open University.

Colditz, G.A., Willett, W.C., Hunter, D.J., Stamper, M.J., Manson, J.E., Hennekens, C.H. and Rosner, B.A. (1993) 'Family history, age, and risk of breast cancer. Prospective data from the Nurses' Health Study', *Journal of the American Medical Association* 270: 338–43.

Coney, S. (1995) *The Menopause Industry*, London: The Women's Press.

Coope, J. (1996) *The Menopause: A Positive Guide to Coping with the Change*, London: Vermillion.

Copeland, J. Bughaigis, M.A. and Schumm, W.R. (1984) 'Relationship characteristics of couples married 30 years or more: a fourth sample replication', *Lifestyles* 7, 2: 107–15.

Copper, B. (1988) *Over the Hill – Reflections on Agism Between Women*, Freedom, CA: The Crossing Press.

Corbin, J. and Strauss A. (1988) *Unending Work and Care: Managing Chronic Illness At Home*, San Francisco: Jossey Bass.

Coupland, J., Coupland, N. and Grainger, K. (1991) 'Intergenerational discourse: contextual versions of ageing and elderliness', *Ageing and Society* 11: 189–208.

Crompton, R. (1997) *Women and Work in Modern Britain*, Oxford: Oxford University Press.

——(ed.) (1999) *Restructuring Gender Relations and Employment. The Decline of the Male Breadwinner*, Oxford: Oxford University Press.

Crompton, R. and Harris, F. (1998) 'Explaining women's employment patterns: "orientations to work" revisited', *British Journal of Sociology* 49:118–36.

Cross, S. and Lovett, J. (1994) 'Women's collective meanings of menopause: a content analysis', *Journal of Women and Aging* 6, 1/2: 187–212.

Cumming, E. and Henry, W. (1961) *Growing Old: The Process of Disengagement*, New York: Basic Books.

Curtis, Z. (1989) 'Older women and feminism: don't say sorry', *Feminist Review* 31: 143–7.

Dalley, G. (1996) *Ideologies of Caring: Rethinking Community and Collectivism*, 2nd edn, London: Macmillan.

D'Arcy, P. (1979) *Song for Sarah*, London: Lion.

Davidson, K. (1999) *Gender, Age and Widowhood: How Older Widows and Widowers Differently Realign their Lives*, unpublished PhD thesis, University of Surrey.

Davies, C. (1995) *Gender and the Professional Predicament in Nursing*, Buckingham: Open University Press.

——(1998) 'Caregiving, carework and professional care', in A. Brechin, J. Walmsley, J. Katz and S. Peace (eds) *Care Matters: Concepts, Practice and Research in Health and Social Care*, London: Sage.

Davis, D.L. (1989) 'The Newfoundland change of life: insights into the medicalization of menopause', *Journal of Cross-Cultural Gerontology* 4: 49–73.

Dearing, R. (1997) *Higher Education in the Learning Society, Report of the National Committee,* The Dearing Report, Main Report, Norwich: HMSO.

Deem, R. (1980) 'Introduction, women, work and schooling: the relevance of gender', in R. Deem (ed.) *Schooling for Women's Work*, London: Routledge and Kegan Paul.

Department of Employment (1992) 'Women and the labour market: results from the 1991 Labour Force Survey', *Employment Gazette* September: 433–59.

Dex, S. (1987) *Women's Occupational Mobility: A Lifetime Perspective*, London: Macmillan.

Dickson, F.C. (1991) 'The best is yet to be: research on long-lasting marriages', in J. T. Wood and S. Duck (eds) *Under-Studied Relationships in Later Life*, Thousand Oaks, CA: Sage.

Dickson, G. (1993) 'Metaphors of menopause', in J.C. Callahan (ed.) *Menopause: A Mid-life Passage*, Bloomington, IN: Indiana University Press.

Di Gregorio, S. (1986) 'Growing old in twentieth century Leeds', unpublished PhD thesis, London School of Economics.

Doty, P., Jackson, M. and Crown, W. (1998) 'The impact of female caregivers' employment status on patterns of formal and informal eldercare', *The Gerontologist* 38: 331–41.

Edwards, R. (1993) *Mature Women Students: Separating or Connecting Family and Education,* London: Taylor & Francis.

Eisenstein, H. (1984) *Contemporary Feminist Thought*, Sydney: Allen and Unwin.

Elias, P. and Gregory, P. (1994) *The Changing Structure of Occupations and Earnings in Great Britain, 1975–1990,* Employment Department Research Series No. 27, Sheffield: Department of Employment.

Equal Opportunities Commission (1992) *Women and Men in Great Britain 1992*, London: HMSO.

Erikson, E. (1980) *Identity and the Life Cycle: A Reissue*, New York: W.W. Norton.

——(1982) *The Life Cycle Completed*, New York: Norton.

Estes, C. (1979) *The Aging Enterprise*, San Francisco: Jossey Bass.

——(1993) 'The aging enterprise revisited', *The Gerontologist* 33: 292–8.

Evandrou, M. (1995) 'Employment and care, paid and unpaid work: the socio-economic position of informal carers in Britain', in J. Phillips (ed.) *Working Carers: International Perspectives on Working and Caring for Older People*, Aldershot: Avebury.

——(ed.) (1997) *Baby Boomers: Ageing in the 21st Century*, London: Age Concern England.

Evandrou, M. and Winter, D. (1992) *Informal Carers and the Labour Market in Britain*. Welfare State Discussion Paper no. 89, STICERD (Suntory–Toyota International Centre for Economics and Related Disciplines), London: London School of Economics and Political Science.

Evans, J. (1995) *Feminist Theory Today: an Introduction to Second-wave Feminism*, London: Sage.

Evers, H. (1981) 'Care or custody? The experiences of women patients in long-stay geriatric wards', in B. Hutter and G. Williams (eds) *Controlling Women: The Normal and the Deviant*, London: Croom Helm.

Featherstone, M. and Hepworth, M. (1990) 'Images of ageing', in J. Bond and P. Coleman (eds) *Ageing in Society*, London: Sage.

——(1991) 'The mask of ageing and the postmodern lifecourse', in M. Featherstone, M. Hepworth and B.S. Turner (eds) *The Body, Social Process and Cultural Theory*, London: Sage.

Ferraro, K. (1984) 'Widowhood and social participation in later life', *Research on Aging* 6: 451–68.

Finch, J. (1995) 'Responsibilities, obligations and commitments', in I. Allen and I. Perkins (eds) *The Future of Family Care for Older People*, London: HMSO.

Finch, J. and Mason, J. (1993) *Negotiating Family Responsibilities*, London: Routledge.

Firestone, S. (1971) *The Dialectic of Sex*, London: Jonathan Cape.

Fisher, M. (1994) 'Man-made care: community care and older male carers', *British Journal of Social Work* 24: 659–81.

Flint, M. and Samil, R.S. (1990) 'Cultural and subcultural meanings of the menopause', in M. Flint, F. Kronenberg and W. Utian (eds) *Multidisciplinary Perspectives on Menopause*, New York: New York Academy of Science.

Ford, J. and Sinclair, R. (1987) *Sixty Years On: Women Talk About Old Age*, London: Women's Press.

Fredriksen, K. and Scharlach, A. (1997) 'Caregiving and employment: the impact of workplace characteristics on role strain', *Journal of Gerontological Social Work* 28, 4: 3–21.

Frick, M. (1972) *All the Days of His Dying*, London: Allison and Busby.

Friedan, B. (1993) *The Fountain of Age*, London: Jonathan Cape.

Fry, C.L. and Gavrin, L. (1987) 'American after lives: widowhood in community context', in H.Z. Lopata (ed.) *Widows: North America*, Durham, NC: Duke University Press.

Gannon, L.R. (1999) *Women and Aging: Transcending the Myths*, London: Routledge.

Garner, J.D. and Mercer, S.O. (eds) (1989) *Women as they Age: Challenge, Opportunity and Triumph*, New York: Haworth Press.

Gee, E.M. and Kimball, M.M. (1987) *Women and Aging*, Toronto: Butterworths.

Genevay, B. and Katz, R. (eds) (1990) *Countertransference and Older Clients*, Newbury Park, CA: Sage.

Gerike, A.E. (1990) 'On gray hair and oppressed brains', *Journal of Women and Aging* 2, 2: 35–46 (special issue on Women, Aging and Ageism).

Gibson, D. (1996) 'Broken down by age and gender – "the problem of old women" redefined', *Gender and Society* 10: 433–48.

Giddens, A. (1991) *Modernity and Self-Identity: Self and Society in the Late Modern Age*, Cambridge: Polity Press.

Gilhooly, M. and Redpath, C. (1984) 'Employment and community care of the physically and mentally impaired elderly', unpublished final report to the Scottish Office, Home and Health Department.

Gilligan, C. (1982) *In A Different Voice: Psychological Theory and Women's Development*, Cambridge, MA: Harvard University Press.

Ginn, J. and Arber, S. (1995) 'Pension penalties: the gendered division of occupational welfare', *Work, Employment and Society* 19: 469–97.

Ginsburg, J. (1992) 'The menopause', in J. George, and S. Ebrahim (eds) *Health Care for Older Women*, Oxford: Oxford University Press.

Glaser, B. and Strauss, A. (1971) *Status Passage*, London: Routledge and Kegan Paul.

Glendenning, F. and Battersby, D. (1990) 'Why we need Educational Gerontology and education for older adults: a statement of first principles,' in F. Glendenning and K. Percy (eds) *Ageing, Education and Society*, Keele: Association for Education Gerontology.

Glendenning, F. and Percy, K. (1998) 'Editorial', *Education and Ageing* 13, 3: 205–12.

Goffman, E. (1969) *The Presentation of Self in Everyday Life*, Harmondsworth: Penguin.

Goode, W. (1960) 'A theory of role strain', *American Sociological Review* 25: 483–96.

Granville, G. (1992) 'The role of health visitors with older women – issues of gender and ageism', unpublished MA dissertation, Keele University.

Graveling, M. (1989) *Combining Work with Care. A Survey to Assess the Needs of Carers at Work*, Great Yarmouth: Anglia Harbours Trust.

Green, S. (1991) 'A two faced society', *Nursing Times* 13 November: 30–1.

Greene, R.R. (1986) 'Countertransference issues in social work with the aged', *Journal of Gerontological Social Work* 9, 3: 79–88.

Greer, G. (1991) *The Change: Women, Ageing and the Menopause*, London: Hamish Hamilton.

Griffiths, F. (1995a) 'Women's decisions about whether or not to take hormone replacement therapy: influence of social and medical factors', *British Journal of General Practice* 45: 477–80.

——(1995b) 'Women's health concerns: is the promotion of hormone replacement therapy for prevention important to women?' *Family Practice* 12:54–9.

Griffiths, M. (1998) *Educational Research for Social Justice: Getting Off the Fence*, Buckingham: Open University Press.

Gubrium, J. (1995) 'Taking stock', *Qualitative Health Research* 5, 3: 267–69.

Gullette, M. (1997) 'Menopause as magic marker', in P. Komesaroff, P. Rothfield and J. Daly (eds) *Reinterpreting Menopause*, New York: Routledge.

Gutmann, D. (1987) *Reclaimed Powers: Towards a New Psychology of Men and Women in Later Life*, New York: Basic Books.

Hagestad, G. and Neugarten, B. (1985) 'Age and the life course', in R. Binstock and E. Shanas (eds) *Handbook of Aging and the Social Sciences*, 2nd edn, New York: Van Nostrand Reinhold.

Hajnal, J. (1972) *The Student Trap,* Harmondsworth: Penguin.

Hakim, C. (1993) 'The myth of rising female employment', *Work, Employment and Society* 7: 97–102.

——(1996) *Key Issues in Women's Work,* London: Athlone Press.

——(1998) 'Developing a sociology for the twenty-first century: preference theory', *British Journal of Sociology* 49:137–43.

Hampshire, S. (1962) 'A ruinous conflict', *New Statesman,* 4 May: 652–3.

Harding, S. (1991) *Whose Science? Whose Knowledge? Thinking from Women's Lives,* Milton Keynes: Open University Press.

Harrop, A. (1990) *The Employment Position of Older Women in Europe: a Demographic Profile,* London: Age Concern Institute of Gerontology.

Heath, M. (1976) 'Pre-retirement Courses as an Instrument of Self-fulfilment in Retirement', unpublished MEd thesis, University of Manchester.

Help the Aged (1994) *Help the Aged Seniorcare Survey,* London: Help the Aged.

Hemmings, S. (1985) *A Wealth of Experience: the Lives of Older Women,* London: Pandora Press.

Hen Co-Op (1993) *Growing Old Disgracefully – New Ideas for Getting the Most Out of Life,* London: Piatkus.

——(1996) *Disgracefully Yours – More Ideas for Getting the Most Out of Your Life,* London: Piatkus.

Her Majesty's Government (1999) *Caring About Carers: A National Strategy for Carers,* London: HM Government.

Herman, S. (1994) 'Marital satisfaction and the elderly', *Gerontology and Geriatrics Education* 14, 4: 69–79.

Heron, A. (1961) *Preparation for Retirement: Solving New Problems,* London: NCSS.

Hess, B. and Soldo, B. (1985) 'Husband and wife networks', in W. Sauer and R. Coward (eds) *Social Support Networks and Care of the Elderly,* New York: Springer.

Hochschild, A. (1983) *The Managed Heart: Commercialisation of Human Feeling,* Berkeley, CA: University of California Press.

Holmes, J. (1993) *John Bowlby and Attachment Theory,* London: Routledge.

Holmes, T.H. and Rahe, R.H. (1967) 'The social readjustment rating scale', *Journal of Psychosomatic Research* 11: 213–18.

hooks, b. (1984) *Feminist Theory from Margin to Centre,* Boston: South End Press.

Hooyman, N. and Gonyea, J. (1995) *Feminist Perspectives on Family Care: Policies for Gender Justice,* Thousand Oaks, CA: Sage.

Hope, K. and Bernard, M. (1992) *A Deceptive Appearance: An Exploration of Ageism,* learning package and video, STAG (Stockport, Tameside and Glossop) College of Nursing: Stockport.

Hughes, B. and Mtezuka, M. (1992) 'Social work and older women: where have older women gone?', in M. Langan and L. Day (eds) *Women, Oppression and Social Work – Issues in Anti-discriminatory Practice,* London: Routledge.

Humm, M. (1989) *The Dictionary of Feminist Theory,* London: Harvester Wheatsheaf.

Hunt, A. (ed.) (1988) *Women and Paid Work: Issues of Equality,* Basingstoke: Macmillan.

Hunter, S. and Sundel, M. (1989) 'Introduction: an examination of key issues concerning midlife', in S. Hunter and M. Sundel (eds) *Midlife Myths*, Newbury Park, CA: Sage Publications.

Hutton, W. (1996) *The State We're In*, London: Vintage.

Itzin, C. and Newman, S. (1995) *Gender, Culture and Organisational Change: Putting Theory Into Practice*, London: Routledge.

Jamieson, A. and Victor, C. (1997) 'Theory and concepts in social gerontology', in A. Jamieson, S. Harper and C. Victor (eds) *Critical Approaches to Ageing and Later Life*, Buckingham: Open University Press.

Jenkins, H. and Allen, C. (1998) 'The relationship between staff burnout/ distress and interactions with residents in two residential homes for older people', *International Journal of Geriatric Psychiatry* 13: 466–72.

Jenkins, R. (1996) *Social Identity*, London: Routledge.

Jerrome, D. (1981) 'The significance of friendship for women in later life', *Ageing and Society* 1: 175–97.

——(1990) 'Intimate relationships', in J. Bond and P. Coleman (eds) *Ageing and Society*, London: Sage.

——(1991) 'Frailty and friendship', *Journal of Cross-Cultural Gerontology* 5: 51–64.

——(1993) 'Intimacy and sexuality amongst older women', in M. Bernard and K. Meade (eds) *Women Come of Age – Perspectives on the Lives of Older Women*, London: Edward Arnold.

Jewish Women in London Group (1989) *Generations of Memories: the Voices of Jewish Women*, London: Women's Press.

Johnson, D., White, L., Edwards, J. and Booth, A. (1986) 'Dimensions of marital quality: towards methodological and conceptual refinement', *Journal of Family Issues* 7: 31–49.

Johnson, J. and Bytheway, B. (1993) 'Ageism: concept and definition', in J. Johnson and R. Slater (eds) *Ageing and Later Life*, London: Sage.

Johnson, M. (1978) 'That was your life', in V. Carver and P. Liddiard (eds) *An Ageing Population*, Sevenoaks: Hodder and Stoughton.

Jones-Porter, E. (1994) 'The life world of older widows: the context of the lived experience', *Journal of Women and Aging* 7, 4: 31–46.

Joseph, A. and Hallman, B. (1996) 'Caught in the triangle: the influence of home, work and elder location on work–family balance', *Canadian Journal of Aging* 15: 393–413.

Joshi, H. (1995) 'The labour market and unpaid caring: conflict and compromise', in I. Allen and S. Perkins (eds) *The Future of Family Care for Older People*, London: HMSO.

Jung, C.G. (1968) *Analytical Psychology: Its Theory and Practice*, New York: Vintage Books.

Kaufert, P. (1982) 'Myths and the menopause', *Sociology of Health and Illness* 4, 2: 141–65.

Kaye, H. (1999) 'Angst about grey matter', *Times Higher Educational Supplement*, 5 November: 10.

Keating, N. and Cole P. (1980) 'What do I do with him 24 hours a day?', *The Gerontologist* 20: 84–9.

Keith, P.M., Dobson, C.D., Goudy, W.J. and Powers. E.A. (1981) 'Older men: occupation, employment status, household involvement and well-being', *Journal of Family Issues* 2: 336–49.

Keith, P.M., Schafer, R.B. and Wacker, R. (1992) 'Outcomes of equity/inequity among older spouses', *International Journal of Aging and Human Development* 36, 3: 187–97.

Kemp, S. and Squires, J. (eds) (1997) *Feminisms*, Oxford: Oxford University Press.

Kimmel, D. (1990) *Adulthood and Aging*, London: John Wiley.

Klass, D. (1996) 'The deceased child in the psychic and social worlds of bereaved parents during the resolution of grief', in D. Klass, P.R. Silverman and S.L. Nickman (eds) *Continuing Bonds*, Washington: Taylor & Francis.

Klass, D., Silverman, P.R. and Nickman. S.L. (eds) (1996) *Continuing Bonds*, Washington: Taylor & Francis.

Komesaroff, P., Rothfield, P. and Daly, J. (eds) (1997) *Reinterpreting Menopause: Cultural and Philosophical Issues*, New York: Routledge.

Kübler-Ross, E. (1970) *On Death and Dying*, London: Tavistock.

Kwok Wei Leng (1997) 'Menopause and the great divide: biomedicine, feminism and cyborg politics', in P. Komesaroff, P. Rothfield and J. Daly (eds) *Reinterpreting Menopause: Cultural and Philosophical Issues*, New York: Routledge.

Labouvie-Vief, G. (1994) 'Women's creativity and images of gender', in B.F. Turner and L.E. Troll (eds) *Women Growing Older*, Newbury Park, CA: Sage.

Laczko, F. and Phillipson C. (1991) *Changing Work and Retirement*, Milton Keynes: Open University Press.

Laslett. P. (1989) *A Fresh Map of Life*, London: Weidenfeld and Nicholson.

Latimer, J. (1997) 'The dark at the bottom of the stairs: performance and participation of hospitalised older people', *Medical Anthropology Quarterly* 15, 2: 31.

Lawler, S. (1996) 'Motherhood and identity', in T. Cosslett *et al.* (eds) (1996) *Women, Power and Resistance – An Introduction to Women's Studies*, Buckingham: Open University Press.

Lawrence, R., Tennstedt, S. and Assman, S. (1998) 'Quality of caregiver–care recipient relationship: does it offset negative consequences of caregiving for family caregivers?', *Psychology and Aging* 13: 150–8.

Layder, D. (1993) *New Strategies in Social Research*, Cambridge: Polity Press.

Levinson, D.J., Darrow, D.N., Klein, E.B., Levinson, M.H. and McKee, B. (1978) *The Seasons of a Man's Life*, New York: Alfred A. Knopf.

Lewis, J. and Meredith, B. (1988) *Daughters Who Care – Daughters Caring for Mothers At Home*, London: Routledge.

Lieberman, M.A. (1994) 'Must widows wear black: growth beyond grief', unpublished manuscript cited in H.Z. Lopata (1996) *Current Widowhood, Myths and Realities*, Newbury Park, CA: Sage.

Lieberman, M.A. and Tobin, S.S. (1983) *The Experience of Old Age: Stress, Coping and Survival*, New York: Basic Books.

Lock, M. (1993) *Encounters with Aging: Mythologies of Menopause in Japan and North America*, Berkeley: University of California Press.

Lopata, H.Z. (1973) *Widowhood in an American City*, Cambridge, MA: Schenkman.

——(1987) *Widows: North America*, Durham, NC: Duke University Press.

——(1996) *Current Widowhood, Myths and Realities*, Newbury Park, CA: Sage.

Love, S. (1997) *The Hormone Dilemma: Should you take HRT?*, New York: Thorsons.

MacDonald, B. and Rich, C. (1984) *Look Me in the Eye: Old Women, Aging and Agism*, San Francisco: Spinsters Book Company.

MacDonald, M. (1980) 'Socio-cultural reproduction and women's education', in R. Deem (ed.) *Schooling for Women's Work*, London: Routledge and Kegan Paul.

Machin, L. (1980) 'Living with Loss', unpublished research report, Lichfield: Lichfield Diocese.

Mackie, F. (1997) 'The left hand of the goddess: the silencing of menopause as a bodily experience of transition', in P. Komesaroff, P. Rothfield and J. Daly (eds) *Reinterpreting Menopause*, New York: Routledge.

MacKinnon, C. (1989) *Towards a Feminist Theory of the State*, Cambridge, MA: Harvard University Press.

McLaughlin, E. (1994) 'Legacies of caring: the experiences and circumstances of ex-carers', *Health and Social Care* 2: 241–53.

Main, M. (1991) 'Metacognitive knowledge, metacognitive monitoring, and singular (coherent) vs multiple (incoherent) model of attachment: findings and direction for future research', in C.M. Parkes, J. Stevenson-Hinde and P. Marris (eds) *Attachment Across the Life Cycle*, London: Routledge.

Marris, P. (1958) *Widows and Their Families*, London: Routledge and Kegan Paul.

——(1974) *Loss and Change*, London: Routledge and Kegan Paul.

——(1982) 'Attachment and society', in C.M. Parkes and J. Stevenson-Hinde (eds) *The Place of Attachment in Human Behaviour*, London: Tavistock.

Marrone, M. (1998) *Attachment and Interaction*, London: Jessica Kingsley.

Martin, E. (1993) *The Woman in the Body: A Cultural Analysis of Reproduction*, Buckingham: Open University Press.

Martin, J. and Roberts, C. (1984) *Women and Employment: A Lifetime Perspective*, London: HMSO.

Martin, M.C., Block, J.E., Sanchez, S.D., Arnaud, C.D. and Beyene, Y. (1993) 'Menopause without symptoms: the endocrinology of menopause among rural Mayan Indians', *American Journal of Obstetrics and Gynecology* 168: 1839–45.

Martin-Matthews, A. (1991) *Widowhood in Later Life*, Toronto: Butterworths.

Martin-Matthews, A. and Rosenthal, C. (1992) 'Structural contexts of work and eldercare', Paper presented at the American Orthopsychiatric Association Meeting. New York.

Mason, J. (1987) 'A bed of roses? Women, marriage and inequality in later life', in P. Allat *et al.* (eds) *Women and the Life Cycle: Transitions and Turning Points*, London: Macmillan.

——(1996) *Qualitative Researching*, London: Sage.

Matthews, S. (1979) *The Social World of Old Women*, San Diego: Sage.

Meade, K. and Walker, J. (1989) 'Gender equality: issues and challenges for preretirement education', *Educational Gerontology* 15: 171–85.

Merrill, B. (1999) *Gender, Change and Identity: Mature Women Students in Universities*, Aldershot: Ashgate.

Merrill, D. (1997) *Caring for Elderly Parents. Juggling Work, Family and Caregiving in Middle and Working Class Families*, Westport: Auburn House.

Miller, B. (1987) 'Gender and control among spouses of the cognitively impaired', *The Gerontologist* 27: 447–53.

Miller, B. and Cafasso, L. (1992) 'Gender difference in caregiving: factor or artefact', *The Gerontologist* 32: 498–507.

Mills, M. (1999) 'Using the narrative in dementia care' in J. Bornat (ed.) *Biographical Interviews: The Link Between Research and Practice*, London: Centre for Policy on Ageing with the Open University.

Minkler, M. (1996) 'Critical perspectives on ageing: new challenges for gerontology', *Ageing and Society* 16: 467–87.

Minkler, M. and Estes, C.L. (eds) (1991) *Critical Perspectives on Aging: the Political and Moral Economy of Growing Old*, Amityville, NY: Baywood Publishing.

Mitchell, J. and Oakley, A. (eds) (1986) *What is Feminism?*, Oxford: Basil Blackwell.

Moen, P., Robison, J. and Fields, V. (1994) 'Women's work and caregiving roles: a life course approach', *Journal of Gerontology: Social Sciences* 49, 4: S176–186.

Moi, T. (1989) 'Feminist, female, feminine', in C. Belsey and J. Moore (eds) *Feminist Reader: Essays in Gender and the Politics of Literary Criticism,* London: Macmillan.

Moody, H.R. (1992) *Aging: Concepts and Controversies*, London: Sage.

Moore, B. and Kombe, H. (1991) 'Climacteric symptoms in a Tanzanian community', *Maturitas* 13, 229–34.

Moore, P. (1986) *Disguised – A True Story*, Waco, TX: Word Incorporated.

Morgan, D.L. (1989) 'Adjusting to widowhood – do social networks make it easier?', *The Gerontologist* 29: 101–7.

Murphy, B., Schofield, H. and Nankervis, J. (1997) 'Women with multiple roles: the emotional impact of caring for ageing parents', *Ageing and Society* 17: 277–91.

Neal, M., Chapman, N., Ingersoll-Dayton, B. and Emlen, A. (1993) *Balancing Work and Caregiving for Children, Adults and Elders,* Newbury Park: Sage.

Neugarten, B. (ed.) (1968) *Middle Age and Aging*, Chicago: The University of Chicago Press.

——(1977) 'Personality and aging', in J.E. Birren and K.W. Schaie (eds) *Handbook of the Psychology of Aging*, New York: Van Nostrand Reinhold.

Neugarten, B. and Datan, N. (1973) 'Sociological perspectives on the lifecourse', in P.B. Baltes and K.W. Schaie (eds) *Life-span Developmental Psychology*, New York: Academic Press.

Neugarten, B., Moore, J.W. and Lowe, J.C. (1965) 'Age norms, age constraints and adult socialisation', *American Journal of Sociology* 70: 701–17.

Nieboer, A.P., Lindenberg, S.M., Ormel, J. (1995) 'Phase-differences in the consequences of bereavement for the well-being of elderly men and women', paper presented at the European Congress of Gerontology, Amsterdam, 30 August–2 September.

Nield, S. and Pearson, R. (1992) *Women Like Us*, London: Women's Press.

Nolan, M., Grant, G. and Keady, J. (1996) *Understanding Family Care*, Buckingham: Open University Press.

Norwood, C. (1943) *Curriculum and Examinations in Secondary Schools: Report of the Committee of the Second School Examinations Council*, London: Board of Education.

Oakley, A. (1974) *The Sociology of Housework*, London: Martin Robertson.

——(1981) 'Interviewing women: a contradiction in terms', in H. Roberts (ed.) *Doing Feminist Research*, London: Routledge.

O'Bryant, S. (1988) 'Self differentiated assistance in older widows' support systems', *Sex Roles* 19: 91–106.

Onyx, J., Leonard, R. and Reed, R. (1999) *Revisioning Aging: Empowerment of Older Women*, New York: Peter Lang Publishing.

OPCS (Office of Population Censuses and Surveys) (1992) *General Household Survey*, London: HMSO.

——(1995) *General Household Survey*, London: HMSO.

Open University (1995) 'The caring responsibilities of Open University staff', in *Carers in Employment: A report on the Development of Policies to Support Carers at Work*, London: The Princess Royal Trust for Carers.

Opie, A. (1994) 'The instability of the caring body: gender and caregivers of confused older people', *Qualitative Health Research* 4: 31–50.

Palo-Stoller, E. (1992) 'Gender differences in experiences of caregiving spouses'; in J.W. Dwyer and R.T. Coward (eds) *Gender, Families and Elder Care*, Newbury Park, CA: Sage.

Parker, G. (1990) *With Due Care and Attention: A Review of Research on Informal Care*, 2nd edn, London: Family Policy Studies Unit.

——(1992) 'Counting care: numbers and types of informal carers', in J. Twigg (ed.) *Carers: Research and Practice*, London: HMSO.

——(1993) *With This Body: Caring and Disability in Marriage*, Buckingham: Open University Press.

——(1994) *Where Next for Research On Carers?*, Leicester University: Nuffield Community Care Studies Unit.

Parker, G. and Lawton, D. (1990) *Different Types of Care, Different Types of Carer: Evidence from the General Household Survey*, London: HMSO.

Parkes, C.M. (1972) *Bereavement: Studies of Grief in Adult Life*, Harmondsworth: Penguin.

——(1986) *Bereavement*, 2nd edn, London: Tavistock Publications.

——(1991) 'Attachment, bonding, and psychiatric problems after bereavement in adult life', in C.M. Parkes, J. Stevenson-Hinde and P. Marris (eds) *Attachment Across the Life Cycle*, London: Routledge.

——(1993) 'Bereavement as a psychosocial transition: processes of adaptation to change', in M.S. Stroebe, W. Stroebe and R.O. Hansson (eds) *Handbook of Bereavement*, New York: Cambridge University Press.

Parkes, C.M. and Weiss, R.S. (1983) *Recovery from Bereavement*, New York: Basic Books.

Parsons, K. (1997) 'The male experience of caregiving for a family member with Alzheimer's disease', *Qualitative Health Research* 7: 391–407.

Parton, N. (1996) 'Social work, risk and "the blaming system"', in N. Parton (ed.) *Social Theory, Social Change and Social Work*, London: Routledge.

Pascall, G. and Cox, R. (1993) *Women Returning to Higher Education*, Buckingham: The Society for Research into Higher Education and Open University Press.

Pavalko, E. and Artis, J. (1997) 'Women's caregiving and paid work: causal relationships in late mid-life', *Journal of Gerontology: Social Sciences* 4 July: 170–9.

Peace, S. (1986) 'The forgotten female: social policy and older women', in C. Phillipson and A. Walker (eds) *Ageing and Social Policy*, Gower: Aldershot.

Penning, M. (1998) 'In the middle: parental caregiving in the context of other roles', *Journal of Gerontology: Social Sciences* 53B, 4: S188–97.

Percy, K. (1990) 'The future of educational gerontology: a second statement of first principles', in F. Glendenning and K. Percy (eds) *Ageing, Education and Society,* Keele: Association for Education Gerontology.

Phillips, J. (1991) 'Working caregivers: care review and productivity report', unpublished paper, University of East Anglia, Norwich.

——(1994) 'The employment consequences of caring for older people', *Health and Social Care in the Community*, 2: 143–52.

Phillipson, C. (1982) *Capitalism and the Construction of Old Age,* London: Macmillan.

——(1998) *Reconstructing Old Age: New Agendas in Social Theory and Practice*, London: Sage.

Phillipson, C. and Strang, P. (1983) *The Impact of Pre-Retirement Education: A Longitudinal Evaluation,* Keele: Department of Adult Education, University of Keele.

Pickard, S. (1994) 'Life after a death: the experience of bereavement in South Wales', *Ageing and Society* 14, 191–217.

Pihlblad, C.T. and Adams, D.L. (1972) 'Widowhood, social participation and life satisfaction', *Aging and Human Development* 3: 323–31.

Pringle, K. (1995) *Men, Masculinities and Social Welfare*, London: University College London.

Pruchno, R.A. and Resch, N.L. (1989) 'Husbands and wives as caregivers: antecedents of depression and burden', *The Gerontologist* 29: 159–65.

Ramsey, D. (1994) 'Carers at work. A survey of informal care responsibilities among social work staff in Fife regional council', unpublished paper, Fife Regional Council.

Raphael, B. (1984) *The Anatomy of Bereavement*, London: Unwin Hyman.

Ray, R. (1996) 'A post-modern perspective on feminist gerontology', *The Gerontologist* 36: 674–80.

Rees, C. (1991) 'Social workers, old women and female carers', *Social Work Monographs*, Norwich: University of East Anglia.

Reinharz, S. (1986) 'Friends or foes: gerontological and feminist theory', *Women's Studies International Forum* 9: 503–14.

——(1992) *Feminist Methods in Social Research*, New York: Oxford University Press.

Reitz, R. (1987) *Menopause: A Positive Approach*, London: Unwin Paperbacks.

Ribbens, J. (1989) 'Interviewing – an "unnatural situation"?', *Women's Studies International Forum* 2: 579–92.

Rich, C. (1984) 'Aging, ageism and feminist avoidance', in B. MacDonald and C. Rich (eds) *Look Me in the Eye*, London: The Women's Press.

Richards, L., Carmel, S. and Davies, N. (eds) (1997) *Intermission: Women's Experience of Menopause and Mid-life*, Melbourne: Oxford University Press.

Riley, M.W. and Riley, Jr, J.W. (1999) 'Sociological research on age: legacy and challenge', *Ageing and Society* 19: 123–32.

Rollins, B.C. and Feldman, H. (1970) 'Marital satisfaction over the family life cycle', *Journal of Marriage and the Family* 3, 2: 20–8.

Rosenblatt, P.C. (1993) 'Grief: the social context of private feelings', in M.S. Stroebe, W. Stroebe and R.O. Hansson (eds) *Handbook of Bereavement*, New York: Cambridge University Press.

——(1996) 'Grief that does not end', in D. Klass, P.R. Silverman and S.L. Nickman (eds) *Continuing Bonds*, Washington: Taylor & Francis.

Rosenthal, C., Martin-Matthews, A. and Matthews, S. (1996) 'Caught in the middle? Occupancy in multiple roles and help to parents in a national probability sample of Canadian adults', *Journal of Gerontology: Social Sciences* 51B, 6: S274–83.

Rosik, C.H. (1989) 'Impact of religious orientation in conjugal bereavement amongst older adults', *International Journal of Aging and Human Development* 28: 251–60.

Rossi, A. (1986) 'Sex and gender in an ageing society', *Daedalus* 111: 141–69.

Rossi, I. (1995) 'An assessment of employer sponsored initiatives for assisting employees who are caring for elderly dependants in The Netherlands and the UK', unpublished MA dissertation, University of Bath.

Rowe, D. (1994) *Time on Our Side – Growing in Wisdom, Not Growing Old*, London: HarperCollins.

Rowbotham, S. (1973) *Woman's Consciousness, Man's World*, Harmondsworth: Penguin.

Rubery, J. and Fagan, C. (1994) 'Occupational segregation: plus ça change…?', in R. Lindley (1994) (ed.) *Labour Market Structures and Prospects for Women*, London: Equal Opportunities Commission.

Sable, P. (1989) 'Attachment, anxiety and the loss of a husband', *American Journal of Orthopsychiatry* 59: 550–56.

Sarnoff Schiff, H. (1977) *The Bereaved Parent*, New York: Souvenir Press.

Scharlach, A. and Boyd, S. (1989) 'Caregiving and employment: results of an employee survey', *The Gerontologist* 29: 382–7.

Schram, R. (1979) 'Marital satisfaction over the family life cycle: a critique and proposal', *Journal of Marriage and the Family* February: 7–12.

Schulz, R. (1990) 'Theoretical perspectives on caregiving: concepts, variables and methods', in D.E. Biegel and A. Blum (eds) *Aging and Caregiving: Theory, Research and Policy*, Newbury Park, CA: Sage.

Schut H.A.W., Stroebe M.S. and Vanden Bout J. (1997) 'Intervention for the bereaved: gender differences in the efficacy of two counselling programmes', *British Journal of Clinical Psychology* 36: 63–72.

Seddon, D. (1998) 'Caregiving and employment: a qualitative study of carers of people with dementia', unpublished PhD thesis, Bangor, University of Wales.

Seibold, C.I (1997) 'The body in mid-life', in L. Richards, C. Seibold and N. Davis (eds) *Intermission: Women's Experience of Menopause and Mid-life*, Melbourne: Oxford University Press.

Shapiro, J. (ed.) (1989) *Ourselves Growing Older: Women Ageing with Knowledge and Power*, London: Fontana.

Sheehy, G. (1994) *The Silent Passage: Menopause*, London: HarperCollins.

——(1995) *New Passages. Mapping your Life Across Time*, New York: Ballantine Books.

——(1997) *New Passages*, London: HarperCollins.

Sidell, M. (1995) *Health in Old Age – Myth, Mystery and Management*, Buckingham: Open University Press.

Siegel, R.J. (1990) 'We are not your mothers: report on two groups for women over sixty', in E.R. Rosenthal (ed.) *Women, Aging and Agism*, New York: Haworth Press.

Silverman, P. (1987) 'Widowhood as the next stage in the life course', in H.Z. Lopata (ed.) *Widows: North America*, Durham, NC: Duke University Press.

Silverman, P. and Klass, D. (1996) 'Introduction: what's the problem', in D. Klass, P.R. Silverman and S.L. Nickman (eds) *Continuing Bonds*, Washington: Taylor & Francis.

Slater, R. (1995) *The Psychology of Growing Old*, Buckingham: Open University Press.

Sontag, S. (1978) 'The double standard of ageing', in V. Carver and P. Liddiard (eds) *An Ageing Population*, London: Hodder and Stoughton.

Sporakowski, M.J. and Axelson, L.V. (1984) 'Long term marriage: a critical review', *Lifestyles of the Elderly* 7, 2: 76–93.

Steier, F. (ed.) (1991) *Research and Reflexivity*, London: Sage.

Stephens, M. and Townsend A. (1997) 'Stress of parent care – positive and negative effects of women's other roles,' *Psychology and Aging* 12: 376–86.

Stevenson, O. (1989) *Age and Vulnerability*, London: Edward Arnold.

Stohs, J. (1994) 'Alternative ethics in employed women's household labor', *Journal of Family Issues* 15: 550–61.

Stroebe, M. (1992) 'Coping with bereavement: a review of the grief work hypothesis', *Omega* 26: 19–42.

Stroebe, M., Gergen, M., Gergen, K. and Stroebe, W. (1996) 'Broken hearts or broken bonds?', in D. Klass, P.R. Silverman and S.L. Nickman (eds) *Continuing Bonds*, Washington: Taylor & Francis.

Stroebe, M.S., Stroebe, W. and Hansson, R.O. (eds) (1993) *Handbook of Bereavement*, New York: Cambridge University Press.

Sugarman, L. (1986) *Life-Span Development: Concepts, Theories and Interventions*, London: Methuen.

Sutherland, G. (1984) *Ability, Merit and Measurement. Mental Testing and English Education 1880–1940*, Oxford: Clarendon Press.

Szinovacz, M. (1980) 'Female retirement: effects on spousal roles and marital adjustment', *Journal of Family Issues* 1: 423–40.

——(ed.) (1982) *Women's Retirement: Policy Implications of Recent Research*, Beverly Hills, CA: Sage.

Tamir, L.M. and Antonucci, T.C. (1981) 'Self perception, motivation and social support through the life course', *Journal of Marriage and the Family* February: 151–60.

Thomas, K. (1990) *Gender and Subject in Higher Education*, Buckingham: Society for Research into Higher Education (SRHE) and Open University Press.

Thone, R.R. (1992) *Women and Aging – Celebrating Ourselves*, New York: Harrington Park Press.

Thornton, P. and Tozer, R. (1995) *A Meeting of Minds: Older People as Research Advisors*, York: Social Policy Research Unit.

Tinker, A. (1994) 'Future prospects for family care and employment', unpublished paper given at the European Foundation for the Improvement of Living and Working Conditions and The German Government conference on Working and Caring, Bonn.

Tong, R. (1989) *Feminist Thought: A Comprehensive Introduction*, Boulder, CO: Westview.

Torrie, M. (1975) *Begin Again*, London: JM Dent and Sons.

Tout, K. (1995) 'An aging perspective on empowerment', in D. Thursz, C. Nusberg and J. Prather (eds) *Empowering Older People*, London: Cassell.

Townsend, P. (1981) 'The structured dependency of the elderly: a creation of social policy in the twentieth century', *Ageing and Society* 1: 5–28.

——(1986) 'Ageism and social policy', in C. Phillipson and A. Walker (eds) *Ageing and Social Policy: A Critical Assessment*, Aldershot: Gower Publishing Group.

Tseelson, E. (1995) *The Masque of Femininity*, London: Sage.

Turner, B.F. and Troll, L.E. (eds) (1994) *Women Growing Older – Psychological Perspectives*, Thousand Oaks, CA: Sage.

Twigg, J. (ed.) (1992) *Carers: Research and Practice*, London, HMSO.

——(1999) 'Carework as bodywork', unpublished paper given at the Conference of the British Society of Gerontology, September, Bournemouth.

Twigg, J. and Atkin, K. (1994) *Carers Perceived: Policy and Practice in Informal Care*, Buckingham: Open University Press.

Ungerson, C. (1987) *Policy is Personal – Sex, Gender and Informal Care*, London: Tavistock.

——(1997) 'Payment for caring – mapping a territory', in C. Ungerson and M. Kember (eds) *Women and Social Policy. A Reader*, 2nd edn, London: Macmillan.

Vickers, M. (1997) 'Separating hype from hope in HRT', *Medical Research Council News* 73: 21–24.

Walby, S. (1997) *Gender Transformations*, London: Routledge.

Walker, A. (1981) 'Towards a political economy of old age', *Ageing and Society* 1: 73–94.

——(1982) 'Dependency and old age', *Social Policy and Administration* 16, 2: 115–35.

——(1987) 'The poor relation: poverty among older women', in C. Glendenning and J. Millar (eds) *Women and Poverty in Britain*, Hemel Hempstead: Harvester Wheatsheaf.

——(1992) 'Conceptual perspectives on gender and family caregiving', in J.W. Dwyer and R.T. Coward (eds) *Gender, Families and Elder Care*, Thousand Oaks, CA: Sage.

——(1993) *Age and Employment: Policies, Attitudes and Practice*, London: Institute of Personnel Management Research Series.

Wallhagen, M. (1992) 'Caregiving demands: their difficulty and effects on the well being of elderly caregivers', *Scholarly Inquiry for Nursing Practice* 6, 2: 111–27.

Walter, T. (1996) 'A new model of grief: bereavement and biography', *Mortality* 1: 1.

Watanabe Greene, R. and Field, S. (1989) 'Social support coverage and the well-being of elderly widows and married women, *Journal of Family Issues* 10: 33–51.

Wenger, G.C. (1990) 'Elderly carers: the need for appropriate intervention', *Ageing and Society* 10, 2: 197–219.

West, C. (1993) 'The new cultural politics of difference', in S. During (ed.) *The Cultural Studies Reader,* London: Routledge.

West, L. (1996) *Beyond Fragments*, London: Taylor & Francis.

Whatmore, K. (1990) *Care to Work,* National Carers Survey, vol. 1. London: Opportunities for Women.

Willis, S. and Reid, J. (eds) (1999) *Life in the Middle: Psychological and Social Development in Middle Age*, San Diego: Academic Press.

Wilson, R. (1966) *Feminine Forever*, London: W.H. Allen.

——(1995) *Understanding HRT and the Menopause*, London: Which? Consumers' Association.

Wolf, D. and Soldo, B. (1994) 'Married women's allocation of time to employment and care of elderly parents', *Journal of Human Resources* 29: 1259–76.

Woodward, K. (1991) *Aging and Its Discontents*, Bloomington, IN: Indiana University Press.

Worcester, N. and Whatley, M. (1992) 'The selling factor of HRT: playing on the fear factor', *Feminist Review* 41: 1–24.

Worden, W. (1991) *Grief Counselling and Grief Therapy,* 2nd edn, London: Tavistock/Routledge.

Young, R. and Kahana, E. (1989) 'Specifying caregiver outcomes: gender and relationship aspects of caregiving strain', *The Gerontologist* 29, 5: 660–6.

Yow, V. (1994) *Oral History*, London: Sage.

Zarit, S. (1989) 'Do we need another 'stress and caregiving' study?', *The Gerontologist* 29: 147–8.

Zarit, S., Todd, P.A. and Zarit, J.M. (1986) 'Subjective burden of husbands and wives as caregivers: a longitudinal study', *The Gerontologist* 26: 260–7.

Zedek, S. and Mosier, K. (1990) 'Work in the family and employing organisation', *American Psychologist* 45: 240–51.

Zita, J. (1993) 'Heresy in the female body: the rhetorics of menopause', in J. Callahan (ed.) *Menopause, A Mid-life Passage*, Bloomington, IN: Indiana University Press.

Index

DATE DUE

GAYLORD

PRINTED IN U.S.A.